Overcoming Your Smoking Habit

The aim of the **Overcoming** series is to enable people with psychologically based disorders to take control of their own recovery program. Each title, with its specially tailored program, is devised by a practising clinician using the latest techniques of cognitive behavioral therapy – techniques which have been shown to be highly effective in changing the way patients think about themselves and their problems.

The series was initiated in 1993 by Peter Cooper, Professor of Psychology at Reading University and Research Fellow at the University of Cambridge in the UK whose original volume on overcoming bulimia nervosa and binge-eating continues to help many people in the USA, the UK and Europe.

Other titles in the series include:

Overcoming Anger and Irritability
William Davies

Overcoming Anorexia Nervosa
Christopher Freeman

Overcoming Anxiety
Helen Kennerley

Bulimia Nervosa and Binge-Eating
Peter J. Cooper

Overcoming Childhood Trauma
Helen Kennerley

Overcoming Compulsive Gambling
Alex Blaszczynski

Overcoming Depression (new revised edition)
Paul Gilbert

Overcoming Low Self-Esteem
Melanie Fennell

Overcoming Mood Swings
Jan Scott

Overcoming Panic
Derrick Silove & Vijaya Manicavasagar

Overcoming Social Anxiety and Shyness
Gillian Butler

Overcoming Traumatic Stress
Claudia Herbert & Anna Wetmore

All titles in the series are available by mail order from Constable Robinson Ltd. Please ring 020 8741 3663 for details.
www.constablerobinson.com

OVERCOMING YOUR SMOKING HABIT

*A self-help guide using
cognitive behavioral techniques*

David F. Marks

ROBINSON
London

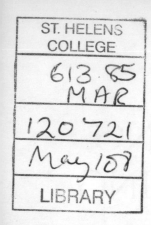
Constable & Robinson Ltd
3 The Lanchesters
162 Fulham Palace Road
London W6 9ER
www.constablerobinson.com

First published in the UK by Robinson,
an imprint of Constable & Robinson Ltd 2005

A copy of the British Library Cataloguing in
Publication Data is available from the British Library.

ISBN 1-84529-067-4

2 4 6 8 10 9 7 5 3 1

Important Note
This book is not intended to be substitute for medical advice or treatment.
Any person with a condition requiring medical attention should consult
a qualified medical practitioner or suitable therapist.

Printed and bound in the EU.

Contents

Contents

Introduction

Why cognitive behavior therapy?

You may have picked up this book uncertain as to why a psychological therapy such as cognitive behavioral therapy could help you overcome your smoking habit. Smoking is a physical addiction, you might think. Cognitive behavioral therapy is for people who have psychological problems, and that's not me. In fact although CBT was developed initially for the treatment of depression, the techniques this therapy uses have been found to be extremely effective for a wide range of problems including compulsive gambling and drug and alcohol addiction. So what is CBT and how does it work?

In the 1950s and 1960s a set of techniques was developed, broadly collectively termed 'behavior therapy'. These techniques shared two basic features. First, they aimed to remove symptoms (such as anxiety) by dealing with those symptoms themselves, rather than their deep-seated underlying historical causes (traditionally the focus of psychoanalysis, the approach developed by Sigmund Freud and his followers). Second, they were techniques, loosely related to what laboratory psychologists were finding out about the mechanisms of learning, which could potentially be put to the test, or had already been proven to be of practical value to sufferers. The area where these techniques proved of most value was in the treatment of anxiety disorders, especially specific phobias (such as fear of animals or heights) and agoraphobia, both notoriously difficult to treat using conventional psychotherapies.

After an initial flush of enthusiasm, discontent with behavior therapy grew. There were a number of reasons for this, an important one of which was the fact that behavior therapy did not deal with the internal thoughts which were so obviously central to the distress that patients were experiencing. In particular, behavior therapy proved inadequate when it came to the treatment of depression. In the late 1960s and early 1970s a treatment was developed specifically for depression called 'cognitive therapy'. The pioneer in this enterprise was an American psychiatrist, Professor Aaron T. Beck, who developed a theory of depression which emphasized the importance of people's depressed styles of thinking. He also specified a new form of therapy. It would not be an exaggeration to say that Beck's work has changed the nature of psychotherapy, not just for depression but for a range of psychological problems.

The techniques introduced by Beck have been merged with the techniques developed earlier by the behavior therapists to produce a therapeutic approach which has come to be known as 'cognitive behavior therapy'. This therapy has been subjected to the strictest scientific testing; and it has been found to be a highly successful treatment for a significant proportion of cases of depression. However it has become clear that specific patterns of thinking are associated with a range of psychological problems and that treatments which deal with these styles of thinking are highly effective. So, effective cognitive behavioral treatments have been developed for anxiety disorders, like panic disorder, generalized anxiety disorder, specific phobias and social phobia, obsessive compulsive disorders, and hypochondriasis (health anxiety), as well as for other conditions such as compulsive gambling, alcohol and drug addiction, and eating disorders like bulimia nervosa and binge-eating disorder. Indeed, cognitive behavioral techniques have a wide application beyond the narrow categories of psychological disorders: they have been applied effectively, for example, to helping people with low self-esteem those with marital difficulties or weight problems, and those who wish to give up smoking.

The starting point for CBT is that the way we think, feel, and behave are all intimately linked; and changing the way we think about ourselves, our experiences, and the world around us, changes the way we feel and what we are able to do. So, by helping a depressed person identify and challenge their automatic depressive thoughts, a route out of a cycle of depressive thoughts and feelings can be found. Similarly, addictive behaviour, such as that associated with smoking, is driven by a nexus of thoughts, feelings and behaviours; and CBT, as you will discover from this book, by providing a means for the addictive behaviour to be brought under cognitive control, enables habitual responses to be undermined and a different kind of life to be possible.

Although effective CBT treatments have been developed for a wide range of problems, they are not widely available; and when people try to help themselves they often make matters worse. In recent years the community of cognitive behavior therapists has responded to this situation. What they have done is to take the principles and techniques of specific cognitive behavior therapies for particular problems and represent them in self-help manuals. These manuals specify a systematic program of treatment which the individual sufferer is advised to work through to overcome their difficulties. In this way, the cognitive behavioral therapeutic techniques of proven value are being made available on the widest possible basis.

Self-help manuals are never going to replace therapists. Many people will need individual treatment from a qualified therapist. It is also the case that, despite the widespread success of cognitive behavioral therapy, some people will not respond to it and will need one of the other treatments available. Nevertheless, although research on the use of cognitive behavioral self-help manuals is at an early stage, the work done to date indicates that for a very great many people such a manual will prove sufficient for them to overcome their problems without professional help.

Many people suffer silently and secretly for years. Sometimes appropriate help is not forthcoming despite their efforts to find it. Sometimes they feel too ashamed or guilty to reveal their problems to anyone. For many of these people the cognitive behavioral self-help manual will provide a lifeline to recovery and a better future.

Professor Peter Cooper
The University of Reading, 2004

Preface

Welcome to *Overcoming Your Smoking Habit*. If you are a smoker and would like to quit, this book is for you. Rarely can psychology be directly applied to a life-threatening situation and actually help to save lives! But, in this case, it really can do that. If you are a smoker, reading this book could not only help to save your life, it could contribute to a healthier and longer life as well. It could also save you a large amount of money – which will go up in smoke unless you overcome the habit.

I have spent thirty years developing more successful ways of helping smokers overcome the habit. My research has brought me into contact with people from all backgrounds, cultures and occupations going through the process of quitting. Many have reported feelings of empowerment, self-control and deep satisfaction in achieving what had previously seemed impossible – giving up smoking. Nothing can give a smoker a greater boost to his or her self-esteem than to give up the smoking habit successfully.

My interest in smoking began in the 1970s when I was a smoker myself and experienced the unpleasant effects of addiction. While living in the USA, I switched to low-tar cigarettes; I was inhaling more deeply and I started getting headaches as a consequence. So I decided to quit smoking, and discovered for myself how difficult it was. I was living in New Zealand in the late 1970s, where I developed the Isis Stop Smoking Programme with Paul Sulzberger. The key methods were drawn from cognitive behavior therapy (CBT) and the programme was delivered in five group therapy sessions over a period of eight days. The Isis Programme is still running today, and independent research carried out by the Heylen Research Centre showed that the Isis Programme produced very exciting results.

In the mid-1980s I returned to the UK, as Head of the School of Psychology at Middlesex Polytechnic in North London. I redesigned the cognitive therapy programme as the QUIT FOR LIFE or QFL Programme. The busy London lifestyle was very different from that of the more laidback New Zealanders, so I needed to find a more efficient approach that did not require as many group sessions. The therapy was converted to a self-help pack, including a book and an audio tape that could be used with only a small number of sessions with a therapist – or even none at all. The new self-help version was published by the British Psychological Society and is still available in public libraries in the UK and Ireland.

Smoking is one of the most addictive and harmful habits that anyone can acquire. This book aims to give you the best possible chance of overcoming your smoking habit. The methods described are based on psychological theory and research, and have been evaluated with hundreds of smokers in randomized controlled trials. Many thousands of smokers have already successfully overcome their smoking habit using these methods. If you use the procedures described, with commitment and perseverance, you will be able to overcome your smoking habit for ever. You too can be a calm and confident non-smoker.

Overcoming Your Smoking Habit is in three stages. In Part One I discuss the psychology of smoking and of quitting. I introduce the powerful methods of cognitive behavior therapy (CBT), why they work, and how they can be applied by you to overcome your smoking habit once and for all. It will help you to think about what you do when you smoke, why you do it, and what smoking really means to you.

Part Two will take you from being an addicted smoker on day 1 through to a new life as a non-smoker 7 to 10 days later. This really is a new beginning, a brand new life the best possible way to improve your health.

In Part Three I show you how to *prevent relapse* and *maintain your non-smoking permanently*. If you follow all of the procedures described, you have an excellent chance of becoming a permanent non-smoker.

Why You Should Quit Smoking

Quitting smoking is, in all probability, the most important thing you can do to improve your health. If you can quit smoking:

- You will live longer and live a healthier life.
- You will significantly reduce your chance of having a heart attack, stroke, or cancer.
- If you are pregnant, quitting smoking will improve your chances of having a healthy baby.
- The people you live with, especially your children, will be healthier.
- You will save a lot of extra money to spend on other things.

How This Book Can Help You

However keen you are to start, before the process of quitting can be started, you need to read Part One. This introduces the main ideas behind this particular approach to smoking addiction, and to the psychological theory and research that supports CBT as the best available method for quitting smoking. To gain maximum results, don't be tempted to skip any sections of this book. If you follow the procedures as directed, on a day-by-day basis, you will be able to stop smoking easily and permanently.

This book describes about thirty different procedures all of which have proven helpful to thousands of people in the past. Nobody can predict which particular methods you will find the most useful – smokers show large differences in the way they respond to each method. However, by offering you a wide range of different procedures, the CBT Programme gives you an excellent chance of success. And, believe it or not, you can actually enjoy the experience of quitting smoking! You can learn a lot about yourself and the potential you have to change the things that you do that you'd like to change. Drinking, eating, shopping, lounging, watching the television, gambling – anything done to excess can become a problem. Smoking is a habit which seems difficult to change, but it can be brought under control easily and permanently by applying this systematic psychological programme.

The book can be used as a stand-alone, self-help method of quitting or it can be combined with the treatment offered by your local health service providers. In the UK, the National Health Service system for helping people to quit smoking is based on a method called 'withdrawal-oriented therapy' (WOT), which was developed at the Institute of Psychiatry in London. The approach focuses on smoking as a form of drug addiction and helps to maintain abstinence during the initial withdrawal discomfort over the first few weeks. It also uses medication to provide relief from the withdrawal symptoms, and group sessions to give extra support. In the US, help for smokers is given by a large variety of organizations, both public and private. The quality is variable and hard to predict. In most other places in the world, the local health services for smokers are generally very basic and offer little help in the form of techniques for overcoming the smoking habit. Essentially the smoker is left to his or her own devices, which in the end means willpower. The UK health care system even claims to 'make your willpower more powerful'. As you know already, willpower alone is never enough. The smoker needs skills for learning to control smoking in a systematic way. CBT can usefully complement the basic WOT system to provide a total treatment package, taking you through the transition from full-blown addiction to a state of non-smoking.

The CBT system described in this book is called the 'Quit For Life Programme'. The Quit For Life or 'QFL' Programme as mentioned earlier was originally published by the British Psychological Society and has been thoroughly evaluated in scientifically controlled trials. If you want to find out more about the results of the formal clinical trials, details are in two of my own articles, which you will find in the Useful References section on p. 197. In order to obtain the maximum benefit from this book, please follow the instructions in Part Two step by step, until you reach your 'D-Day' or Quit Day.

CBT is different from many other forms of psychological treatment. The typical method of quitting tries to build up the smoker's motivation to the point where the smoker is meant to stop smoking *instantaneously* purely by the strength of his or her will. Using willpower, perhaps combined with special drugs, the smoker is meant to make a permanent transformation. So the smoker is expected to think and feel completely differently purely by making a decision to do so.

In this CBT programme you learn different feelings and thoughts about smoking over a period of 7 to 10 days, using cognitive behavior therapy. We know that a habit built up over many years or even decades cannot disappear overnight. You need time to change, and time to recondition your thoughts and feelings. This cannot be done by a miraculous decision to do so.

Yet this is what the traditional methods expect of you: you tell yourself to stop by a certain date and it will happen. Now if that could be achieved permanently that really would be a miracle. Haven't you tried that already? And haven't you discovered that miracles like that simply do not happen? No wonder the results from such traditional 'willpower' procedures generally are so poor.

Overcoming your smoking habit will take time. Not necessarily a very long time, but a week to ten days. This book tells you exactly what you need to do in an easy step-by-step programme. To aid your success, there are two simple Golden Rules.

Two Golden Rules

Golden Rule 1:
Smoke a cigarette every time you feel like one.

Golden Rule 2:
Do your homework – practise the CBT exercises
whenever you feel like smoking.

The exercises provided in Part Two give you all the ammunition you need to destroy your smoking habit once and for all. The experience with thousands of smokers before you shows that the procedures are simple but highly effective when consistently applied.

Before You Begin

Here are some relevant factors that you should take into account before you begin the process of quitting:

Timing

Timing is of the essence. At certain times, circumstances may preclude making such a major change. For example, if you are in the process of changing jobs, have recently lost your job, or are going through a separation or divorce, or have just suffered a bereavement or other trauma, this is definitely not a suitable time to attempt to stop smoking.

It takes a period of consolidated effort to be able to quit smoking successfully. If you are going through other major changes at the same time, you won't be able to manage the necessary effort to quit smoking as well. In those cases, it would be better to wait until things settle down before embarking upon this programme.

Another easy-to-arrange factor is the day of week when you begin the programme. Experience suggests that it is better to make progress over the main part of the week first, then to tackle the weekend. For many people the weekend is very different from their usual Monday to Friday routine, so the weekend will need some special planning when you are in the middle of quitting smoking.

The best day to begin the programme is a Tuesday. By starting then you will be able to reduce your cigarette consumption to manageable proportions by the weekend. You will also avoid the 'Monday Effect', caused by the extra stress and hassle after the more leisurely days of Saturday and Sunday. It's also a good idea to steer clear of weeks ending in long weekends or special occasions such as Christmas, New Year, festivals and holidays, because you need to quit when things are relatively normal and routine. That gives you the best chance to quit smoking.

Motivation

Motivation is a major factor. A smoker's desire to quit waxes and wanes, but the best time for you to quit is when you really want to stop. Simply being persuaded, nagged, or cajoled to do so by another person is definitely not enough. Of course, everybody who cares about you should want you to quit and should encourage and support you while you are doing so. But you have to really want to stop smoking for yourself, not for anybody else: only you can make the conscious decision that now is the time to quit and you're going to do it.

In thinking about your motives, consider three things: your health, your attractiveness, and your wealth. Firstly, your health. The health effects of smoking are well known; they are discussed further in chapter one. Secondly, attractiveness. Smoking may have seemed a cool thing to do when you first started, but nowadays it's stinkingly uncool to smoke. Thirdly, consider your pocket. If you are on a 40-a-day habit, you're literally burning £3,000 per year. Over 25 years, that's £75,000, plus the interest. Think what you could do with that money instead. You probably do not need much more persuading than this.

Working Through the Programme

As you work through the programme, you will need to read one chapter in Part Two of the book every day, for five days. Each chapter will will prepare you to apply the methods over the next 24 hours. Follow the instructions and apply the methods as systematically as you possibly can. Everything you need to eliminate smoking from your life is contained in this programme. All that you need in addition is your personal commitment.

In reading this book stopping smoking is your primary objective. However, the same techniques can be applied to other aspects of your health and lifestyle as well. After you have successfully stopped smoking, you may consider applying these same methods to other areas of your life where you feel you need to make changes, such as eating or drinking.

Summary

- Start the process of quitting when the rest of your life is running on a fairly even course.
- Start the process because you really want to, not because you want to please somebody else. Prepare yourself thoroughly by reading the relevant section of the book the day before you actually need to apply it.
- Start only when you are prepared to really work at it.
- Golden Rule 1 tells you to smoke every time you feel like smoking, right up to your Quit Day. Continue to smoke during the first part of the Programme.
- Golden Rule 2 tells you carry out the CBT exercises whenever you smoke or feel like smoking.

- Enjoy the process of change! Successfully making the changes that you most desire can be very exciting.

I wish you complete success in becoming a happy and successful non-smoker.

Acknowledgements

The author would like to thank Catherine M. Sykes for her assistance and enthusiasm in carrying out the research that enabled the CBT programme described herein, to be evaluated. I also thank Paul Sulzberger who originally developed the ISIS Programme when we were both working at the University of Otago, in New Zealand, and also Kathleen Campbell, David Carter, Lati Haddad, Ian Hodgson and Gillian Pow for their support in researching and developing the therapy. The now defunct Health Education Authority gave permission to reprint extracts from *Enjoy Healthy Eating* (in chapter 9) and *Exercise. Why Bother?* (in chapter 10).

PART ONE

Understanding Your Smoking Habit

Part One of the book discusses the history, behaviour, experience, addiction and treatment of smoking, and new effective ways of quitting. The powerful methods of cognitive behavior therapy are described, including why they work and how they can be applied by you.

Understanding Smoking and Smoking Addiction

How Many People Smoke?

At the start of the twenty-first century, approximately one in four of the adult population is a smoker. Three-quarters admit that they would like to quit the habit. Unfortunately, only 5 to 6 per cent of those who attempt to quit on their own continue to be non-smokers for more than one year. Most relapse within a few days of each attempt at quitting.

There are large gender differences in the way tobacco is used. The World Health Organization (WHO) estimates that 47 per cent of men and 12 per cent of women smoke, including 42 per cent of men and 24 per cent of women in developed countries, and 48 per cent of men and 7 per cent of women in developing countries. Although fewer women are smokers than men, there have been dramatic increases in smoking among women; the gap between men and women in smoking rates is narrowing in most places.

What's in the Smoke?

Tobacco smoke is a lethal cocktail; there are around 600 poisons in every cigarette. Cigarettes contain small quantities of chemicals that are also present in paint stripper, toilet cleaner, lighter fuel, mothballs, gas chambers, and rocket fuel.

According to a 1998 report by the Scientific Committee on Smoking and Health (SCOTH), the tar content of tobacco smoke is the single most important health risk. The SCOTH Report found that tar yields have fallen over the past few decades in all brands. This was achieved in part by a 'cheat' method, in which small air holes were placed in cigarette filters so that when the tar yields are measured they became diluted by the air. The report concluded that any benefits flowing from the increased usage of low-tar brands are offset by an increase in the usage of hand-rolled tobacco, in which tar content is high.

Yields of nicotine in hand-rolling tobacco are higher on average than those from manufactured cigarettes. The amount of nicotine in manufactured cigarettes is not regulated, but yields have tended to fall as tar levels have reduced. However, the new filters have resulted in the presence of extra air mixed in with the smoke. Smokers therefore inhale with a longer and deeper puff to obtain the same amount of nicotine as they used to – so more carbon monoxide is drawn into the smoker's respiratory system, and from the lungs into the bloodstream.

Yields of nitrogen, such as nitric oxide, depend on the type of tobacco and are independent of tar. Nitric oxide is produced by the decomposition of nitrates in tobacco and is inhaled by the smoker. Although inhaled nitric oxide appears to have no direct toxic effect, exhaled nitric oxide (including nitric oxide in side-stream smoke) gradually oxidizes to nitrogen dioxide, which is a respiratory irritant.

What are the Health Effects?

The health effects of smoking have been studied for over one hundred years. The evidence has been collated by health authorities throughout the world. It is one of the best-researched topics in the medical sciences. Even the tobacco industry admits the health risks, albeit in a minimized form. The Centers for Disease Control and Prevention in the US give a useful guide to the health impacts of smoking. Smoking accounts for 440,000 deaths each year in the US and 120,000 deaths in the UK, nearly 1 of every 5 deaths. More deaths are caused each year by tobacco than by all deaths from human immunodeficiency virus (HIV), illegal drug use, alcohol use, motor vehicle injuries, suicides, and murders combined. The risk of dying from lung cancer is at least 22 times higher among men who smoke, and about 12 times higher among women who smoke, compared with those who have never smoked.

In the US there have been no less than 28 Surgeon General's Reports on smoking and health during the period 1964–2004. Tobacco is the leading preventable cause of death in the US, causing more than 440,000 deaths each year and resulting in an annual cost of more than $75 billion in direct medical costs. Nationally, smoking results in almost 6 million years of potential life lost each year. Approximately 80 per cent of adult smokers started smoking before the age of 18. Every day, nearly 4,000 people under the age of 18 try their first cigarette. More than 6.4 million children living today will die prematurely because of their decision to smoke cigarettes.

In 2004, the US Surgeon General Richard H. Carmona released a new report on smoking and health, revealing for the first time that smoking causes diseases in nearly every organ of the body. Published 40 years after the Surgeon General's first report on smoking – which concluded that smoking was a definite cause of three serious diseases – the 2004 report finds that cigarette smoking is conclusively linked to diseases such as leukaemia, cataracts, pneumonia and cancers of the cervix, kidney, pancreas and stomach.

According to the report on average, men who smoke cut their lives short by 13.2 years, and female smokers lose 14.5 years. The economic toll exceeds $157 billion each year in the US – $75 billion in direct medical costs and $82 billion in lost productivity.

In 1964, the Surgeon General's report announced research showing that smoking was a definite cause of cancers of the lung and larynx (voice box) in men and chronic bronchitis in both men and women. Later reports concluded that smoking causes a number of other diseases such as cancers of the bladder, oesophagus, mouth and throat; cardiovascular diseases; and reproductive effects. The 2004 report expanded the list of illness and conditions linked to smoking. The new illnesses and diseases linked to smoking include cataracts, pneumonia, acute myeloid leukaemia, abdominal aortic aneurysm, stomach cancer, pancreatic cancer, cervical cancer, kidney cancer and periodontitis.

Statistics indicate that more than 12 million Americans have died from smoking since the 1964 report of the Surgeon General, and another 25 million Americans alive today will most likely die of a smoking-related illness.

The 2004 report concludes that quitting smoking has immediate and long-term benefits, reducing risks for diseases caused by smoking and improving health in general. 'Within minutes and hours after smokers inhale that last cigarette, their bodies begin a series of changes that continue for years,' Dr Carmona stated. 'Among these health improvements are a drop in heart rate, improved circulation, and reduced risk of heart attack, lung cancer and stroke. By quitting smoking today a smoker can assure a healthier tomorrow.'

Dr Carmona has also said that it is never too late to stop smoking. Quitting smoking at age 65 or older reduces a person's risk of dying of a smoking-related disease by nearly 50 per cent.

Cigarette smoking increases the risk for many types of cancer, including cancers of the lip, oral cavity, and pharynx; oesophagus; pancreas; larynx (voice box); lung; uterine cervix; urinary bladder; and kidney. Rates of cancers related to cigarette smoking vary widely among members of racial/ethnic groups, but are generally highest in African-American men. Cigarette smokers are two to four times more likely to develop coronary heart disease than non-smokers. Cigarette smoking approximately doubles a person's risk for stroke. Cigarette smoking causes reduces circulation by narrowing the blood vessels (arteries), and smokers are more than ten times as likely as non-smokers to develop peripheral vascular disease.

Smoking is associated with a ten-fold increase in the risk of dying from chronic obstructive lung disease. About 90 per cent of all deaths from chronic obstructive lung diseases are attributable to cigarette smoking. Cigarette smoking has many adverse reproductive and early childhood effects, including an increased risk for infertility, pre-term delivery, stillbirth, low birth weight, and sudden infant death syndrome (SIDS). Postmenopausal women who smoke have lower bone density than women who have never smoked. Women who smoke have an increased risk for hip fracture than those who have never smoked.

Smoking is the leading preventable cause of death. The WHO estimates approximately 5 million deaths each year worldwide are caused by tobacco consumption, a figure that is expected to double by 2030. Epidemiological research suggests that 50 per cent of all smokers die as a direct result of their smoking habit. Five hundred million people will die from smoking in the first half of the 21st century. This is many more deaths than occurred in all of the wars of the twentieth century. The vast majority of these deaths will occur in the developing world. Please make sure that *you* are not one of its victims!

Naturally, tobacco smoke does most damage to the person who is actively inhaling. However, those nearby who are breathing second-hand or environmental tobacco smoke (ETS) also are likely to have a higher risk of cancer, heart disease, and respiratory disease, as well as sensory irritation. Scientific evidence suggests that smoking causes the premature death of thousands of non-smokers worldwide. SCOTH commissioned a special review of the impact of smoking and lung cancer. This review analyzed 37 epidemiological studies of lung cancer in women who were life-long non-smokers but lived with smokers. The review found that the women's risk of developing lung cancer was raised by 26 per cent. The analysis also showed that there was a relationship between the risk of lung cancer and the number of cigarettes smoked by a person's partner, as well as the duration over which they had been exposed to their smoke. To quote the report, 'SCOTH members concluded that long term exposure of non-smokers to ETS caused an increased risk of lung cancer which, in those living with smokers, is in the region of 20 to 30 per cent'. The estimated increased risk equates to several hundred extra deaths per year in Britain. The report also concluded that smoking by parents caused acute and chronic middle ear disease in children. Furthermore, it concluded that SIDS, the main cause of post-neonatal death in the first year of life, is associated with exposure to environmental tobacco smoke. The association was judged to be one of cause and effect.

Cigarettes are also the major cause of fires in domestic, industrial and public buildings. Tobacco smoke cannot be controlled by ventilation, air cleaning, or separating smokers from non-smokers. Making public places smoke-free is the only real remedy.

What is Addiction?

Addiction occurs when an individual loses control over an activity or type of behaviour. The activity is usually something that is enjoyable or satisfies a need. However, after the individual loses control and cannot contain the activity within reasonable bounds, the behaviour causes a bad impact on the person's well-being. When the behaviour is ceased, unpleasant physical or mental reactions or 'withdrawal symptoms' occur, including craving.

Smoking is one of the strongest addictions. I have encountered some extreme cases. A young man who worked as a waiter in a wine bar once told me that he got through 6 packs (120 cigarettes!) every day. At first I could not understand this. Each cigarette takes, say, five minutes to smoke. If he smoked them one after the other, that would have meant 600 minutes or 10 hours of smoking every day. However, he explained that he would have several cigarettes alight at any one time, left in ashtrays at different tables, so he could be anywhere in the table area and be close enough to one somewhere in the room and be able to have a puff!

Another smoker told me that she had to set her alarm clock to wake her at 3.30 am every morning so that she could have a cigarette in the middle of the night, to guarantee a decent night's sleep.

Another smoker told me that he smoked almost everywhere he went, including the shower. He kept a cigarette alight in a high-up soap dish so he could take a puff whenever he felt like it. It's like imagining somebody trying to light a wet firework that turns into a very damp squib.

UK TV presenter Dale Winton told the London newspaper *Metro* that he is a 30-a-day man. During an attack of bronchitis, he didn't smoke for eight days. This was an excellent opportunity to quit smoking altogether. However, Dale said that all he could think about was the fact that he wanted to get better – just so he could have a cigarette! Now that's addiction for you.

The fact that you can smoke in so many different circumstances and situations is one of the main reasons smoking is such a difficult habit to break. If smoking could be restricted to only one or two situations, the habit would be much easier to control. But you can smoke in the car, house, bed, street, park, bar and restaurant. Although many more restrictions are now in force in public places, there are still plenty of places available for smoking.

A major breakthrough in learning to control your smoking is to appreciate that every separate situation in which you smoke is a distinct and separate smoking habit. When you realize the truth of this statement, you will be ready to begin the process of quitting in a serious manner. Until then, you will be forced into traditional ways of thinking that smoking is a single habit, not a multitude of habits. The title of this book should really be: *Overcoming Your Smoking Habits*!

How Does It Happen?

The addictiveness of tobacco results from the fact that tobacco contains the drug nicotine. Nicotine is a naturally occurring colourless liquid that turns brown when burned, and smells of tobacco when exposed to air. Since nicotine was first identified in the early 1800s, it has been shown to have a number of complex and unpredictable effects on the brain and the body. Most cigarettes contain 10 milligrams (mg) or more of nicotine. The typical smoker takes in 1 to 2 mg nicotine per cigarette. Nicotine is absorbed through the skin and lining of the mouth and nose, or by inhalation in the lungs. In cigarettes nicotine reaches peak levels in the bloodstream and brain very rapidly, within 7–10 seconds of inhalation. Cigar and pipe smokers, on the other hand, typically do not inhale the smoke, so nicotine is absorbed more slowly through the mucosal membranes of their mouths. Nicotine from smokeless tobacco is also absorbed through the mucosal membranes.

Nicotine is addictive because it activates brain circuits that regulate feelings of pleasure, the 'reward pathways' of the brain. A key chemical involved is the neurotransmitter dopamine which nicotine increases. The acute effects of nicotine disappear in a few minutes; this makes the smoker repeat the dose of nicotine, to maintain the drug's pleasurable effects and prevent withdrawal symptoms.

The cigarette is an efficient and highly engineered drug-delivery system. By inhaling, the smoker can get nicotine to the brain very rapidly with each and every puff. A typical smoker will take 10 puffs on a cigarette during the 5-minute period when the cigarette is lit. Thus, a person who smokes 30 cigarettes daily gets 300 'hits' of nicotine every day. That makes over 100,000 hits a year, or one million hits every ten years! This is why cigarette smoking is so highly addictive. Smoking behaviour is rewarded and reinforced hundreds of thousands or millions of times over the smoker's lifetime.

Using advanced technology, scientists have discovered that an enzyme called monoamineoxidase (MAO) shows a marked decrease during smoking. MAO is responsible for breaking down dopamine. The change in MAO is caused by an ingredient other than nicotine, since we know that nicotine does not dramatically alter MAO levels. The decrease in MAO results in higher dopamine levels, another possible reason why smokers continue to smoke – they need to maintain high dopamine levels to keep high satisfaction levels, which leads to repeated drug use. So the reason you have become addicted to nicotine is that changes have occurred in your brain, so you require more nicotine to prevent withdrawal symptoms and maintain an overall pleasant feeling.

Are Some People More Prone to Addiction?

There is evidence that tobacco is the most addictive drug available. More than 30 per cent of people who try tobacco for the first time develop a dependency on tobacco; for other drugs, this percentage is generally lower. However there are variations in the speed and strength of addiction to nicotine among smokers. One obvious way to explain individual differences in smoking is our genetic makeup. Genetic factors could play a role in several aspects of nicotine addiction, from the tendency to begin smoking, to the chances of quitting. Evidence from behavioural studies, twin studies and molecular genetic research is providing a clearer understanding of the biobehavioural basis for nicotine dependence.

Dr Swan and colleagues have analyzed more than 20 studies of smoking behaviours in monozygotic and dizygotic twins. They found consistent evidence of genetic influences governing the developmental stages of smoking (initiation, maintenance, cessation), and smoking intensity (light to heavy), as well as for level of alcohol consumption.

Dr Ernest Noble and colleagues have reported the discovery of a gene that appears to be associated with alcoholism, the D2 dopamine receptor gene (DRD2). Dr. Noble has conducted studies suggesting that the same gene may also be involved in tobacco addiction, cocaine addiction and obesity. I described above the role of dopamine in nicotine addiction. Two main dopaminergic pathways in the brain are in the area called the *substantia nigra*, which is involved with movement, and the *mesolimbic dopamine system (MDS)*, which is associated with emotion. When alcohol, nicotine, cocaine, or food is ingested, dopamine levels increase in the MDS, increasing reward and pleasure.

Other researchers have looked for evidence of personality differences between people who smoke and non-smokers. However the relationships are fairly weak and it can be concluded that anybody has the potential to become addicted to nicotine.

What Withdrawal Symptoms Can I Expect?

Withdrawal symptoms are physical and mental changes that occur following interruption of drug use. They are normally temporary and require a period of adjustment. The withdrawal symptoms following smoking cessation are many and varied. A list of some of the main ones, together with their duration and prevalence, is given in the table below.

Symptom	Duration	Prevalence
Increased appetite	10 or more weeks	70 per cent
Urges to smoke	Greater than 2 weeks	70 per cent
Depression	Less than 4 weeks	60 per cent
Restlessness	Less than 4 weeks	60 per cent
Poor concentration	Less than 2 weeks	60 per cent
Irritability/aggression	Less than 4 weeks	50 per cent
Night-time awakenings/insomnia	Less than 1 week	25 per cent
Strange smoking-related dreams	Less than 1 week	10 per cent
Constipation	More than 2 weeks	10 per cent
Cough/cold symptoms	Less than 4 weeks	10 per cent
Mouth ulcers	More than 4 weeks	10 per cent
Reduced heart-rate	Long-term	90 per cent
Decreased tremor	Long-term	90 per cent
Increased skin temperature	Long-term	90 per cent
Decreased caffeine metabolism	Long-term	90 per cent
Weight increase (6 kg, 13 lb, average)	Long-term	90 per cent
Dietary preferences	Long-term	90 per cent

• Adapted from West (2004)

Unfortunately, some smokers report increased coughing, throat soreness, chest problems and mouth ulcers during or after quitting. This can deter the smoker from continuing with their attempt to quit, by providing an excuse to smoke again; the symptoms increase the risk of relapse. You must be on your guard against this danger. Chapter eight, in Part Three, gives more details on how you can protect yourself against relapse.

You Have a Better Chance of Being Successful If You Have Help

You can get support in many ways:

- Tell your family, friends, and colleagues that you are going to quit and want their support. Ask them not to smoke around you or leave cigarettes out.
- Talk to your doctor, dentist, nurse, pharmacist, psychologist, or smoking counsellor. Inform them that you are using this book and ask them for their support.
- Get individual, group, or telephone counselling. The more counselling you have, the better your chances are of quitting. Call your local smoking cessation service for information about programmes in your area; they are usually based in local hospitals and health centres.

Another factor is the unpleasant sensation of craving which almost all smokers experience during the first few days or weeks after cessation. There are different ways of reducing the pain of craving. You can prevent craving, lapse and relapse by using a variety of non-medical methods. These methods are described in detail in Chapter eight. They have the advantage that they do not use drugs, have no side effects and can therefore be considered as less risky. They also do not risk a new dependency on a drug in the place of nicotine addiction.

One common reason for restarting the habit is fear of weight gain. Many smokers gain weight when they quit. Eating a healthy diet and staying active are the two ways of dealing with this issue. Don't let weight gain distract you from your goal of quitting smoking. These issues will be discussed in detail in Chapters nine and ten.

Do I Need Medication?

One method to reduce the craving and the risk of relapse is to use medication. Taking nicotine in a safer form is the main option. Nicotine replacement therapy (NRT) can lessen the urge to smoke and remove some of the withdrawal effects. Forms of NRT include chewing gum, transdermal patches, nasal spray, inhalers and pills.

In 2004 researchers reviewed how effective the different forms of NRT were in helping people quitting smoking altogether, or reducing the the amount smoked for a sustained period. The review looked at randomized trials in which NRT was compared to placebo (or no treatment), or where different doses of NRT were compared. The measure used was whether the ex-smokers managed to abstain from smoking for at least six months. Ninety-six trials were reviewed against a control group of people quitting smoking who had not used NRT. The group using NRT were 1.74 times more likely to abstain than those not using NRT.

The reviewers concluded that all of the commercially available forms of NRT (nicotine gum, transdermal patch, the nicotine nasal spray, nicotine inhaler and nicotine sublingual pills/lozenges) are effective as part of a strategy to quit smoking. NRT increases quit rates by approximately one and a half to two times. The effectiveness of NRT appears to be largely independent of the intensity of additional support provided to the smoker.

Another alternative is to take a drug called Zyban or bupropion, which was originally designed as an anti-depressant. If you want to gain any benefit from Zyban, you will need to start taking it 1–2 weeks before you begin this programme. Four randomized studies have compared 12-month cessation rates with placebo. For bupropion 300 mg a day for 7 to 12 weeks, 105 out of 518 smokers (20 per cent) had stopped at 12 months, compared with 34 out of 430 smokers (8 per cent) using placebo. One study directly compared NRT to bupropion and showed that Bupropion was significantly more effective than nicotine patches or placebo. However, more research on buproprion is needed before firm conclusions can be reached.

An issue to be aware of, if you are contemplating using Zyban, is the possibility of side effects. The most common side effects are a dry mouth, insomnia, a change in appetite, agitation and headaches. The most common side effects which cause people to discontinue use of bupropion are shakiness and skin rash. Rarely, bupropion can cause seizures. If you already have epilepsy or an existing seizure disorder, you definitely should NOT take this drug. It is also important to carefully follow your doctor's recommendations about dosage, due to the risk of seizures.

To sum up, the main types of medication that are available to help you quit are:

1 Zyban or Bupropion – available by prescription.
2 Nicotine gum – available over-the-counter.
3 Nicotine inhaler – available by prescription.
4 Nicotine nasal spray – available by prescription.
5 Nicotine patch – available by prescription and over-the-counter.

You can also obtain tablets and lozenges (see page 130).

You need to ask for advice from your doctor and carefully read the information on the package. If you are pregnant or trying to become pregnant, breastfeeding, under the age of 18, smoking fewer than 10 cigarettes per day, or have a medical condition, talk to your doctor or advisor before taking medication.

In using cognitive behavior therapy to quit smoking, it is quite possible that CBT could help you make the necessary changes without any need for a nicotine substitute or other medication. Many hundreds of my clients have successfully quit by using CBT alone. This is one of the major benefits of using CBT – it allows you to overcome your smoking habit without the need for medication. However, you may wish to consider a moderate dosage of NRT in combination with CBT, if you are unable to control your craving in any other way. Further details of NRT are given in Chapter eight.

Can I Use CBT while Receiving Other Treatment?

Local health services generally provide the minimum level of support that should be given to would-be quitters. The training of counsellors who run the smoking cessation services usually does not include CBT. The training is aimed at minimizing the problem of withdrawal by the use of medication. It does not attempt to give psychological support in the form of techniques for quitting. It is not surprising that many smokers treated by the health care system are dissatisfied with the service that they receive. The drop-out rate is very high.

CBT methods can improve the results of any treatment programme. For example, CBT is ideally suited to complement the withdrawal-oriented treatment already being offered. If you enrol for treatment in a smoking clinic, then I would strongly recommend that you apply CBT before you reach your quit day. This will enable you to minimize the drawbacks of using willpower. It will teach you how to control your smoking behaviour in a rational way. It will help to remove the pleasure and satisfaction that is currently being provided by smoking.

For Pregnant Women Only: Can CBT Help Me To Quit Smoking Before I Have My Baby?

Smoking is an important issue for the health of both the mother and the baby. Unfortunately, many women and girls continue to smoke while trying for a baby, with only a minority successfully quitting when they become pregnant. Research has demonstrated that smoking during pregnancy causes health problems for both mothers and babies, such as pregnancy complications, premature birth, low-birth-weight infants, stillbirth, and infant death. Low birth-weight is a leading cause of infant deaths, resulting in more than 300,000 deaths annually in the US.

Pregnant women who smoke are about twice as likely to experience complications such as placenta praevia, a condition where the placenta grows too close to the opening of the uterus. This condition frequently leads to delivery by a Caesarean section. Pregnant women who smoke also are more likely to have placental abruption, where the placenta prematurely separates from the wall of the uterus. This can lead to pre-term delivery, stillbirth, or early infant death.

Pregnant smokers are at a higher risk for premature rupture of membranes before labour begins. This makes it more likely that a smoker will carry her baby for a shorter than normal gestation period and the baby will therefore have a lower birth-weight. Risk for having a baby in the smallest 5 to 10 per cent of birth weights is as high as 2.5 times greater for pregnant smokers. It is therefore essential for you to quit smoking if you are to have the best chance of having a healthy baby. The first trimester is the best time to quit.

CBT is ideally suited to quitting during pregnancy. It is a safe, natural method that minimizes the role of willpower and the use of medication. Ideally, medication should be avoided in pregnancy. Doctors discourage the use of NRT and Zyban during pregnancy, so NRT should only be used as a last resort if CBT fails. The 24-hour NRT patch gives the the foetus even more nicotine than cigarettes do. The effects of nicotine on the later development of the baby remain uncertain.

For Cannabis Users Only: Can I Quit Smoking Tobacco but Continue to Smoke Cannabis?

Many tobacco smokers also smoke cannabis. Cannabis is the most widely used illicit drug. In the UK, Cannabis resin, or 'hash', is often mixed with tobacco in 'roll-ups', or joints. The smoker continues to smoke tobacco because he or she wishes to continue smoking cannabis and thinks it's not possible to do one without doing the other. This link between cannabis use and tobacco is unfortunate. Smoking is the most damaging way of using cannabis, because cannabis gives off three times as much tar and five times more carbon monoxide than average manufactured cigarettes.

Whilst cannabis itself is not addictive, the tobacco or nicotine in the tobacco is very addictive. For someone trying to stop smoking, mixing tobacco and cannabis is a very bad idea. It is possible to smoke or ingest cannabis without mixing it with tobacco.

A New Zealand study of the effects of tobacco and cannabis exposure on lung function in young adults looked at the use of cannabis and tobacco smoking at various ages. The subjects' lung function – the volume of air they could breathe out in one second – was tested. There was evidence of a linear relationship between cannabis use and lung function, daily cigarette smoking affected it even more. So using cannabis in smoked form may not be as safe as is often assumed by users.

Many users think smoking cannabis is safe. However, some studies suggest that smoking pure cannabis is more harmful to lungs than tobacco. A study by the British Lung Foundation found that just three cannabis joints a day cause the same damage as 20 cigarettes. When cannabis and tobacco are smoked together, the effects are dramatically worse. Evidence shows that tar from cannabis cigarettes contains 50 per cent more cancer-causing carcinogens than tobacco.

In the brain, tetrahydocannibinol (THC) activates specific sites (called cannabinoid receptors) in the parts of the brain that influence pleasure, memory, thought, concentration, sensory and time perception, and co-ordinated movement. Puff volume with cannabis is often three or four times higher than with tobacco – in other words, you inhale deeper and hold your breath with the smoke for longer before exhaling. This results in more carbon monoxide and tar entering into the lungs.

Many cannabis smokers become addicted to tobacco purely as a side effect of smoking cannabis. They would not consider themselves principally as tobacco smokers. Practices vary across the world. Over 80 per cent of cannabis users in Britain smoke tobacco, either mixed with cannabis or by itself in cigarettes, when they finally realize they are tobacco addicts. The new smoker associates the high produced by the tobacco and cannabis mix as that from cannabis alone. Unfortunately, tobacco can addict you within a few tries, and new smokers can then feel that they 'need' a joint, not realizing that it is tobacco addiction kicking in. A new cannabis user will soon start smoking tobacco at regular intervals to maintain nicotine levels.

I have tried several times to help regular cannabis users break their nicotine addiction. It failed because they refused to stop smoking cannabis and tobacco together. If you are a regular cannabis user you must either quit using it or change the way you use cannabis if you are to have a good chance of quitting tobacco.

The Case of James

James was a 29-year-old working for an investment bank in the City of London. With degrees in politics and IT, James had taken time out to travel around the world. He was finding his job very stressful and worked long hours. He smoked ten cigarettes a day, Monday to Wednesday: one on his way to work, two during breaks at work and approximately seven in the evening. Thursday to Sunday would be spent in the pub, drinking with friends and smoking about twenty cigarettes a day.

As he approached the age of thirty, James started to think more seriously about his health. He and the friend he lived with decided to quit smoking together. They purchased some nicotine gum. They decided that the first step would be to cut down using the gum. So they used the gum in certain situations. For example, in the evenings after work, James had two cigarettes plus several pieces of gum. During the day at work, he had one cigarette at work and one piece of gum. They managed to cut down their cigarette consumption for ten days. However, they relapsed at the weekend, when they both smoked twenty cigarettes each in a night out in London. They both agreed that the taste of the gum was horrible and that the summer was not a good time to give up smoking, as it was a very sociable time. So they continued to smoke.

The following New Year's Eve, James decided he would quit smoking by 'cold turkey', not using any method except willpower. He had noticed that he had begun to smoke more and was still worried about his health. This time, he quit smoking for one month. However, once more, it was a night spent in the pub that started him smoking again. At first, it was just one a day, but slowly he was back to smoking ten a day during the week and double that at the weekend.

James' friend recommended that he visit a health psychologist. She had heard about a friend who had quit successfully using 'QUIT FOR LIFE'. James felt determined to quit. He was beginning to feel unfit and dreaded the thought of becoming ill due to smoking, something that he felt he should be able to control. He felt very nervous about going to see a psychologist. He had always associated psychologists with mental illness. Nevertheless, he trusted the advice of his friend and turned up for a pre-treatment session with the psychologist. During the session, James' motivation for stopping smoking was identified as related to health reasons. They agreed to set his start day for the following Tuesday, when a treatment session would be held with the psychologist. We will follow James' progress at different stages of this book.

Summary

- Smoking causes more deaths each year than HIV, drug use, alcohol use, accidents, suicides and murders combined. It is a major cause of both cancer and heart disease.
- Nicotine addiction is caused by changes in the reward or pleasure centres of the smoker's brain. Although individual variations exist, everybody who tries a cigarette is at risk of addiction.
- One in four of the adult population smokes. Three-quarters would like to quit but they have only a 5 to 6 per cent chance of lasting a year without returning to smoking.
- Nicotine replacement therapy (NRT) or bupropion (Zyban) are available to support the quitter if needed. NRT substitutes one form of nicotine by another but its dosage can be gradually reduced. However, it is not recommended during pregnancy. The most effective form of treatment is to use CBT and then add NRT to overcome withdrawal. In many cases CBT can work without NRT. CBT enables the smoker to regain control over their behaviour.
- Pregnant women are urged to quit smoking in their first trimester using CBT – that is, using a safe and natural method.
- Quitters who use cannabis are advised not to smoke cannabis, or to ingest it in some other form. Otherwise, for smokers who combine marijuana with tobacco, tobacco smoking is likely to restart, as the smoker returns to the habit of mixing cannabis with tobacco to make a joint.

2

How Cognitive Behavioral Therapy Can Help You Quit Smoking

General Principles

Probably you have tried to quit smoking many times before, and you know how hard it can be. Usually people have to try several times before finally being able to quit. Nicotine is a very addictive drug, more addictive than heroin or cocaine.

Each time you have tried to quit, even though you did not make it, you have learned something about what helps and what hinders you. That knowledge will help you now. One of the main principles of the cognitive behavioral therapy (CBT) approach is that you must learn as much as possible about your smoking habit so that you can learn how to change it. This is the best possible preparation for your first step on the seven-step ladder described below.

1 Getting prepared.
2 Getting support.
3 Removing the reward value and pleasure of smoking.
4 Learning not to respond to smoking triggers.
5 Removing the stress-smoke spiral.
6 Getting medication and using it correctly.
7 Preparing for relapse or difficult situations.

You have the best chances if you progress along each of these steps in turn. This book will give you everything you need to move through these stages. The traditional methods of quitting smoking advocate the use of strong willpower combined with medication. Cognitive behavior therapy is a more advanced and effective approach. It is simple, free, harmless, powerful, and natural. In using CBT you will be using the power of the mind to heal itself, by controlling your behaviour, and changing your experience of pleasure that you gain from smoking. In using CBT, you will be much less reliant or willpower and drugs, both of which have drawbacks.

Willpower is often not available in sufficient amounts to make the changes that you desire. Most smokers are just too weak-willed to quit smoking without other means of help. As a consequence, this may well lead to a visit to the doctor, who will give you medication. To an increasing extent these days, smoking is being treated using drug therapy alone, when a more powerful and natural approach is available using CBT. In many cases, a combination of the two approaches will work best.

Drugs may be used to temporarily remove the cravings and urges that lead to smoking, and they may substitute for the nicotine itself. However, substituting one form of nicotine with another is not a cure. None of the psychological triggers that lead to smoking are removed by drug therapy; as soon, as the NRT is no longer available, the triggers will pull you back to cigarettes. Drugs also have unwanted side effects and may be as addictive as tobacco itself. There is certainly no point in replacing one addiction by another. Medication, if used wisely, can be extremely beneficial. But it works best in combination with techniques that allow you to modify your behaviour: that is, CBT.

In the UK, the National Health Service has not yet adopted CBT for patients who smoke. Lobbying by the pharmaceutical industry swayed our health authorities to adopt a simple drug-based approach. The UK Department of Health advocates CBT for treatment of anxiety and depression, eating disorders and obesity. Yet the Department has adopted the traditional medical model of offering nicotine replacement therapy (NRT) or, another drug, Zyban, as a treatment for smokers.

The medical model is a poor performer when it comes to human behaviour change. Smoking has both physical and psychological aspects. Drugs can address the physical aspects of smoking, but cannot change the psychological aspects. To date, the results from the UK National Health Service system of quitting smoking are disappointing. No objective data has been published on the actual abstinence rates, validated by biochemical markers, either short-term or long-term. All that the statistics show is how many people said that they had quit at four weeks. By their own account almost half (47 per cent) fail to quit by week four of the programme: a disappointing figure given the level of resources. As these results are made public, and policy makers appreciate the limitations of a purely pharmacological approach, alternative methods will come to the fore.

CBT uses the power of the mind to heal and restore the body by modifying excessive, unhealthy and maladaptive behaviours and feelings. Mental processes can change behaviour, thoughts and feelings by setting new goals and plans. CBT is safe, effective, and the best method of quitting smoking available today.

Why Isn't Willpower Enough?

The main reason willpower is not enough is that it is extremely difficult to break an addiction purely because you want to. It doesn't matter how much you try to force yourself to stop smoking because your addiction is a physiological state, similar to hunger. The longer you leave it, the worse it gets. Cravings for nicotine, when you have been unable to smoke for a while, are similar to cravings for food when you're hungry or for water when you are thirsty. The nicotine addiction has created a new bodily need. The root cause of the cravings may be so persistent that they require powerful psychological techniques that have been especially developed to change habits and addictions.

Each and every occasion that you have a smoke is a separate smoking habit. Each set of circumstances in which you smoke contains at least one 'trigger' that sets a whole chain of activity moving. You have learned these chains of behaviour over several months or years. Now you need a system for breaking your smoking chains, for reversing the learning that has gone on over a very long time.

Another reason willpower is not enough is that the body and mind are never fixed in one stable state. There is a constant flux of energy and activity as the individual responds to the changing demands of the environment. When the demands are high the body/mind may lack sufficient resources to deal with these demands. This state is generally referred to as 'stress'. The smoker always responds to stress by smoking. This creates a 'stress-smoke spiral', in which the stress triggers smoking and smoking triggers more stress. The two things serve as triggers for each other, creating a self-perpetuating spiral. It is difficult to escape the spiral without a controlled intervention.

Automatic Programmes

Another way of understanding smoking behaviour is to look at the automatic programmes in your brain that control your everyday activities. Your smoking behaviour is a chain of events that is triggered off without any conscious awareness on your part. Much of the time, you can smoke without even being totally aware of what you are doing. Psychologists refer to this as 'mindlessness'. This means that you have drifted into an automatic state, in which you carry out routine things without any conscious control. Many of our most basic behaviours are of this type, for example walking, standing, sitting, riding a bicycle, driving a car, or even writing or speaking.

Such complex behaviours are controlled by automatic programmes set off in your brain in response to stimuli in the environment. The environment includes both external and internal events. Specialists who become experts in particular skills learn to carry out complicated activities without needing to use any conscious planning or control, for example painting, playing the piano, conducting an orchestra, or swerving a ball into a goal.

The better learned the behaviour, the more automatic it becomes. Think about learning to ride a bicycle. At first the rider can hardly even sit on the saddle without falling off. Every move has to be consciously planned and decided. Then, if somebody supports and guides the bike, while the rider puts their feet on the pedals and starts to pedal, it will be possible to ride the bicycle without falling off. Eventually, the novice can learn to pedal and control the bicycle, and stay balanced without any external help. Then, with more and more practice, he or she can learn to ride the bike smoothly without thinking about each separate action.

A similar process is involved in learning to smoke. At first the novice will find it a very unpleasant and difficult process. The smoke tastes toxic and hot, and the initiate will probably feel sweaty and notice their pulse racing, perhaps even with palpitations. The natural tendency is to cough and choke on the fumes of the tobacco, and it takes a considerable amount of focused attention to continue the puffing activity. With perseverance, the novice can begin to inhale the smoke without coughing. It happens more and more automatically. Nicotine directly affects the brain and, during the first few cigarettes, the reward, reinforcement and addiction processes begins to kick in. The smoker soon becomes tolerant to the unpleasant sensations in their mouth and throat, and cigarettes can be smoked without even noticing unpleasant physiological effects. Eventually, it is satisfying to smoke because the addiction has become stronger and the smoker needs a fix of nicotine to maintain the level of nicotine in the body above a certain level.

Perhaps you can remember your own first cigarette. Can you honestly say that you enjoyed it? If you are honest with yourself, you will probably admit that you hated every second of it. Quite often the initiate is with a friend or two. The initiates put on the bravest of faces while, deep down, longing for the cigarette to be finished and stubbed out. However, this antipathy and need for a 'brave face' doesn't last for long. Nicotine takes over and, before long, you are its slave, with nicotine-controlled smoking chains and automatic programmes ruling your behaviour.

What is CBT?

Because CBT will be new to many readers, I will briefly explain what it is and what it is not.

CBT will enable you to:

- use a set of principles that you can apply to your thinking and beliefs, that will reduce the pleasure and reward value of smoking
- monitor your smoking behaviour, so that you understand when and why it happens
- learn new skills and behaviours, to help prevent you from responding to smoking triggers
- take you off the stress-smoke spiral
- control smoking with a minimum usage of drugs
- control smoking with minimum use of willpower
- lead a normal, healthy life

What CBT is not

CBT is not:

- A form of brain-washing. You do it because you want to do it. It can never happen against your will.
- A form of hypnosis. You carry out CBT in a fully alert, awake state of consciousness.
- Magic. Although the effects can be very impressive, it is not magic, but a natural mental method of controlling your own behaviour.
- A way of increasing your willpower. Your willpower will not be affected by CBT. You may need to use willpower less, but CBT does not increase it.
- A way of controlling the environment. It is you that will change, and the way that you react to the environment, not the environment itself.

Evidence that CBT can help you quit

Smoking is one of the most addictive and dangerous habits that any human being can acquire. It is the most difficult habit to overcome. Rarely can a smoker successfully overcome the habit simply by using power of will. It takes a lot more skill and dogged perseverance than most people possess, as well as sheer hard work. The smoker requires skills and techniques that he or she can have real confidence in. Psychology has a lot to offer in the form of theory, research and practice about behaviour change. Smoking is a very stubborn behaviour to change, but it can be changed and will be changed if the right principles are adopted.

The CBT methods described in this book have been thoroughly tried and tested, not only in the field of smoking but for all kinds of behaviours and experiences – in fact anything that people want to change.

CBT has been tried in various forms by tens of thousands of smokers with results that are among the best on record. Figure 1 shows the dramatic reduction in consumption that was obtained in the original Isis Programme. This reduction curve is based on data collected from 1,000 participants in a 1992 study.

The smoker reduces cigarette consumption gradually over a few days and then quits smoking altogether. Like thousands of others, you can overcome your smoking habit within seven to ten days.

With my colleagues Rumina Dewshi and Catherine Sykes, I ran randomized controlled trials to evaluate the effectiveness of CBT in comparison to a standard health promotion intervention used by the UK National Health System. The results showed that the CBT programme was more than three times more effective than the standard treatment. QFL was evaluated in a randomized controlled trial. The Quit For Life Programme was found to be 3.38 times more cost-effective than the control intervention – many more people quit, using CBT, for a relatively low extra cost.

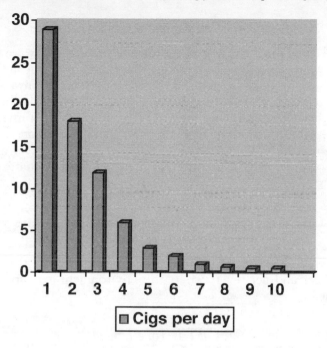

□ **Cigs per day**

CBT uses an empowerment strategy that is designed to put the control of smoking behaviour in your own hands. The techniques are described in detail in Parts Two and Three of this book. Explore your social and psychological environment for cues, motives and symbols that affect your smoking behaviour and experience. Use all of the methods, because the chances of success are increased with the number of methods you choose to employ.

In Part Two, I show you how to reduce your cigarette consumption each day until it reaches zero. While doing this, you will learn how to keep any discomfort down to the minimum. After successfully completing your D-Day, you will be ready for Part Three, which will show how you to maintain your non-smoking on a permanent basis.

Before you begin using the programme, it will be helpful to understand the principles of cognitive behavior therapy.

Principles of CBT

CBT emphasizes the important role of thinking in how we feel and what we do. It is our thinking that causes us to feel and act the way we do. Therefore, if we are experiencing unwanted feelings and behaviours, it is important to identify the thinking that is causing the feelings and behaviours and to learn how to replace this thinking with thoughts that lead to more desirable reactions.

Cognitive-behavioural therapy has the following characteristics:

1. CBT Assumes That Thinking Causes Our Actions and Emotional Responses

If we can change the way we think, we can change the way we feel and act, even when the environment remains the same.

2. CBT is Time-limited

CBT is a brief therapy. It uses a self-discovery method and makes use of 'homework' assignments and exercises.

3. CBT is a Collaborative Effort Between the Therapist and the Client

The author and the reader are co-therapists. I will give you ideas to try out and you will see what works and what doesn't work. We are in this together!

4. CBT is Based on Changing Your Thoughts and Actions

CBT helps people to feel and think and act differently. For example, CBT helps to show you the benefits of jumping off the stress-smoke spiral by learning how to feel calm when confronted with undesirable stress.

5. CBT Uses Self-questioning

CBT encourages you to ask questions of yourself, for example, 'I feel like a smoke every time I have a cup of coffee. How can I stop doing that?'

6. CBT is Structured and Directive

CBT gives you new techniques every day. Specific techniques and concepts are illustrated in each chapter for each day until you stop smoking. CBT focuses on the goals you will set. CBT is directive. CBT tells you *what* to do and *how* to do it.

7. CBT is Based on a Learning Model

CBT is based on the assumption that most emotional and behavioural reactions are learned. Therefore, the goal of therapy is to help you to *unlearn* your unwanted reactions and to learn a new way of reacting. When you understand *how, when and where* you are smoking, you will be able to apply the methods to change your responses.

8. CBT Theory and Techniques Rely on Testing Theories and Making Predictions

The inductive method encourages us to test hypotheses about your behaviour to see if they are correct. You become a scientist about your yourself and your smoking and learn to test theories and to make predictions.

9. Homework is a Central Feature of CBT

If you are to be successful, CBT requires you to practise the techniques in this book.

Three Main Areas

CBT focuses on three main areas:

1. *Cognitive Processes – What We Think*

You will learn methods and ways to change your old thinking patterns and habits. You will train your mind to think and respond differently than you have in the past. There are 30 specific methods and techniques that you will learn to use – and you only need to find several methods that work well for you.

Some effective techniques are:

- Slowing down the smoking process to discover what is going on
- Stopping automatic negative thinking or rationalization
- Learning rational and helpful self-statements that can become permanent and 'automatic'
- Learning to listen to the voice of the new you – the non-smoker. Whose voice do you want to listen to, anyhow? Do you have to listen and believe all of the old lies told to you by your addicted self?
- Focusing: what are you paying attention to?
- Imagery rehearsal: Picturing your new behaviours in the old worn-out situations.
- Self-Imaging: who do you want to be? How do you wish to behave? What kind of a person are you becoming?

2. *Behavioural Processes – What We Do*

This is the part where we put into place new behaviours and remove old ones. You must do this in everyday, real-life situations, not just in your head. This is where CBT can be so powerful. This area is tackled right from the very beginning of the process of quitting and all the way through to the end.

3. Emotional Processes – What We Feel

Smoking is an emotion-related behaviour chain and set of experiences. The emotions set the tone for the behaviours. The thoughts set the agenda. It is important to have some type of relaxation or 'de-stress' strategy. Calmness, confidence and peace are the main goals. You must learn to break the stress-smoke spiral.

The quieter and more relaxed you feel as you make the changes, the more easily the therapeutic process can occur. This calmness and peaceful feeling will let the therapy gently take effect and you will in effect make a new beginning. The focus is on healing, healthiness, and inner peace.

The only way an effective 'cure' for smoking can be achieved is by operating on all three of these levels. CBT does that.

Summary

- One reason why it is so difficult to quit smoking using willpower is that each smoking occasion creates a separate smoking habit. It is very difficult to break the links between smoking and its long-term triggers without using techniques that remove the reward value of smoking.

- The National Health Service in the UK uses a medical model that is basic, as it is oriented purely on minimizing withdrawal symptoms. Withdrawal is an important part of quitting smoking but it is not the total process. To overcome smoking, you need a method that tackles the psychological, emotional and social determinants of smoking, as well the purely physical side of smoking. CBT does this.

- CBT can be used alone, or you can combine it with treatment in the UK National Health Service. CBT tackles the causes of smoking and puts the smoker in charge of their own behaviour. It looks at the thinking that makes a smoker continue with the habit, it looks at the behaviour itself – when, where and why it happens – and it looks at the emotional aspects of smoking.

- You are in charge of your own behaviour, your own thoughts and your own feelings. With CBT, can you be in charge of quitting smoking. You can do it now and you can do it permanently.

PART TWO

How To Stop Smoking

Part Two will guide you through a series of steps that will help you to gradually reduce your smoking in preparation for 'D-Day', the first day in your new life as a non-smoker. For Chapters three to five, each chapter covers one day of the programme. Chapter six deals with Day 4 and the days over the weekend leading up to D-Day. Chapter seven deals with D-Day itself.

Each chapter teaches you new skills and techniques that have been carefully designed to help you successfully reduce and then quit smoking. Table 1 overleaf indicates when the various methods will be introduced in the programme. Use this as a guide to your own participation in the programme. Table 1 gives you a checklist of your personal usage of the different procedures. Tick the methods that you have used each day right up to, and including, your D-Day. Then, when you reach Part Three of the book, check off the procedures that you introduce at that stage also. By the time you have completed the Programme, each of the plus signs should have a tick beside it.

To take Day 1 as an example: by the end of your first 24-hour period in this CBT Programme, you should have used, and ticked under Tuesday's column, Methods 1 to 3. By the end of the second 24-hour period, you should have used, and ticked under Wednesday's column, Methods 1 to 6.

	Method
1	Rubber Band around Pack
2	Record all Smoking on Card
3	Program 1 **(NURD)**
4	Enter Daily Total on Chart
5	Program 2 **(WE STD)**
6	Keep a List of Triggers
7	Program 3 **(EASY)**
8	Meditation
9	Imagery Rehearsal
10	Program 4 **(NOGO)**
11	The Eight Steps and Sensitization
12	Music Therapy (Side 2, Cassette)
13	Win the Argument Game
14	List Personal Benefits of Quitting
15	Plan Your D-Day
16	Try Different Ways of Relaxing
17	Rehearse Positive Programs
18	Increase Activity
19	Distraction
20	Buddy System
21	Willpower
22	Learn Fail-Safe Procedure
23	Develop Eating Control Programme
24	Rules for Snacking
25	Develop Exercise Programme
26	Relapse Prevention
27	Assert Non-Smokers' Rights
28	Deconstruct Tobacco Advertising
29	Develop Time Management Skills
30	Prevent Stress and Strain

	Tues	Wed	Thurs	Fri	Week-end	D-Day	Post D-Day
1	+	+	+	+	+		
2	+	+	+	+	+		
3	+	+	+	+	+		
4	+	+	+	+	+	+	
5		+	+	+	+	+	
6		+	+	+	+	+	
7			+	+	+	+	
8			+	+	+	+	+
9			+	+	+	+	+
10			+	+	+	+	+
11				+	+	+	+
12				+	+	+	+
13				+	+	+	+
14				+	+		+
15				+	+		
16				+	+	+	+
17					+	+	+
18					+	+	+
19					+	+	+
20					+	+	+
21						+	+
22						+	+
23							+
24							+
25							+
26							+
27							+
28							+
29							+
30							+

Please make Day 1 a Tuesday. Your D-Day will be a day carefully chosen by you, 7 to 10 days later. D-Day will be a Monday, Tuesday, Wednesday or a Thursday in the week following your starting date.

Please try all of the methods, as this will give you the best possible chance of success.

3

Day 1: Tuesday – Start Deprogramming Your Mind

Advances in psychology and new approaches to behaviour change have led to powerful psychological therapies that enable people to change their habits and addictions without the need for drugs. Cognitive psychologists, who specialize in the investigation of mental processes, have focused on human memory, imagery, language, and consciousness. Behavioural psychologists have studied learning, conditioning, addiction and habit formation. Cognitive behavior therapy (CBT) is a special application of this knowledge to emotional problems, habits and addictions.

The Human Brain as a Biocomputer

The human brain is a highly sophisticated biological computer or 'biocomputer'. The biocomputer consists of the brain and central nervous system (the hardware) and the programs, which enable the system to process information (the software). The hardware is genetic while the software is acquired through experience. This computer metaphor is useful in understanding how the smoking habit is developed, maintained and eliminated.

Much of our mental activity goes on beneath conscious awareness, and our thoughts, feelings, and behaviour are often controlled by unconscious mental processes. A lot of what we do – including some quite complicated activities such as speaking, shuffling a pack of playing cards, and riding a bicycle – is controlled automatically by hidden mental processes which can be conceptualized as computer programs. These automatic activities are the results of long periods of learning, and all habits and skills are learned behaviours. Once these skills and habits are established, it's almost as if we are operating on automatic pilot. At times, the automatic programming of our behaviour is not entirely to our liking, and we would prefer to behave differently, if we were only able to do so. But the automatic pilot does not always relinquish control when we want it to, and we are left repeating our unwanted behaviour, with little conscious ability to do anything to stop it from happening.

This loss of conscious control has some obvious advantages. Imagine how difficult and tedious life would be if we had to consciously plan every word we spoke, or every movement we made in performing everyday tasks. There would simply be too much to think about, and our ability to co-ordinate our thoughts and actions would quickly break down.

Fortunately, having an automatic pilot does not mean that our conduct is necessarily out of our voluntary control. Even well-ingrained habits can be returned to voluntary control, by systematically breaking them down into their components and making these components more deliberate and voluntary. Eventually, a whole habit or routine can be returned to its original non-automatic state, through a process of relearning. The objective of the CBT approach is to eliminate the automatic nature of smoking, by deliberately influencing the thoughts and feelings that occur before, during, and after smoking.

I suggested above that the mind can be viewed as a highly sophisticated biocomputer. The biocomputer is an extremely complicated device, but having a fine set of hardware is not sufficient to guarantee a sensible result. The human biocomputer needs to be programmed in a sensible and orderly way, if it is to function usefully. The computer metaphor can be applied to the processes of personal development and change. As we grow up and our minds develop, we acquire ways of thinking, behaving, and feeling, through observing and interacting with others. Much of our early behaviour involves trial-and-error learning, with associated rewards and punishments. This is a process of 'conditioning'.

Later, after extensive learning has taken place, our thinking, habits, and emotional reactions become relatively fixed and we operate more predictably – like a computer which has been programmed to process information in particular ways.

Unfortunately, not all of our programming is entirely sensible and rational, and we may end up doing some unhealthy things, such as smoking. Our brains are responsible for everything we think, feel, and do. In the case of a smoker, the brain is programmed by the addiction process to carry out smoking, in the same way that a computer is programmed to carry out automatic functions. When we describe smoking as a 'habit' or 'addiction', we are referring to its automatic, compulsive nature and the way in which a smoker no longer feels any real sense of control over when, where, and how much to smoke. It is therefore quite legitimate to think of the smoking habit as an automatic function of a biocomputer that is programmed to smoke. The same programming is responsible for generating the desire to smoke when no nicotine has entered the body for an hour or two. The programming also generates enjoyable feelings during smoking, especially when the desire to smoke was quite strong beforehand.

Eliminating Automatic Programs

Let's look at a typical smoker aged around 30 years who took up smoking at the age of 14 and smokes an average of just under 25 cigarettes per day. This means that they have smoked a total of 90,400 cigarettes since starting the habit. Assuming an average puff rate of 11 puffs per cigarette and an average of 346 seconds to smoke a cigarette, the typical young smoker will therefore have taken nearly one million puffs and spent the equivalent of 362 days – or just under one year – smoking!

So a regular smoker aged only 30 has spent a whole year of their life smoking. This figure would be even higher for older smokers or those who smoke more than 25 cigarettes per day. The 25-a-day smoker is effectively spending 36.5 days each year smoking – that is, more than one month. And in that time the smoker will have taken 100,000 puffs!

A very sizeable percentage of this smoking activity is carried out without the smoker even thinking about what is going on. Because of its automatic nature, the behaviour must be programmed and controlled by the biocomputer. This programming is acquired during the first few experiences of smoking, which typically occur between the ages of 10 and 15 years.

Programming can be acquired through a number of different means. The most prominent sources of programming are social imitation, peer pressure, advertising, and the addictive effects of nicotine. These factors have probably all contributed in some combination to the mental programming which keeps you smoking. Once smoking has become routine, an addiction to nicotine develops. When this happens, the act of smoking is reinforced by the satisfaction which each new shot of nicotine provides.

Any other stimulus that happens to occur alongside the puff of tobacco smoke (e.g. a sip of coffee) will also be associated with the pleasurable release of dopamine. The more often coffee is drunk at the same time a cigarette is smoked, the more the pairing is reinforced. This will lead to a trigger effect, so having a sip of coffee will automatically lead to smoking.

What you need in order to stop smoking, therefore, are:

- methods for eliminating the programs in your biocomputer which make you want to smoke and enjoy the activity
- new programs that make smoking unpleasant and difficult to perform automatically.

The CBT approach achieves these two goals as efficiently and as permanently as possible by working on the hidden mechanisms which make you think, feel, and behave as a smoker. If you follow the procedures carefully, you will eliminate all desire to smoke. After a few days, cigarettes will give you no satisfaction and smoking them will feel unpleasant.

Motivation

The strength of your motivation is a key factor in successfully overcoming your smoking habit. Think about why you want to give up smoking. Is it because you're worried about your health? Or because the habit is becoming a drain on your finances? Write these reasons down and keep them somewhere handy, so you can look at them when you feel like giving up your efforts to quit smoking.

Positive Thinking

Many of us are limited by our own ideas about what we think we can achieve. This is frequently much less than our true potential. One of the biggest difficulties faced by smokers is the conviction that failure is inevitable.

If you are confident that you will achieve your goal, you will be in a better position to do so. Any lurking self-doubts need to be removed right now. If you believe that your chances of stopping smoking are only slight, that belief will sabotage even the most carefully designed program. Tell yourself that, in seven to ten days, you will be a non-smoker and enjoy life much more than you do now. Become optimistic. Become enthusiastic. Most of all, become confident in your own ability to overcome smoking.

To encourage yourself to think more positively, examine the Progress Chart which is printed in Appendix A. Photocopy it and keep it where you can see it throughout the day. Look at it often: in the mornings when you get up, and last thing at night before you go to bed. Remember that, when you look at this chart, you are seeing the same goals thousands of smokers have already achieved successfully before you. There is absolutely no reason why your progress should be any different!

How CBT Can Work For You

You are embarking upon a tried and tested psychological approach that identifies and removes the triggers for smoking that are unique to you as a smoker.

How can I state this with such confidence? Firstly, research with thousands of smokers has shown that CBT will give you a success rate that is much higher than trying to stop smoking on your own. This CBT approach has been thoroughly evaluated before being released and the results have been independently verified and published in scientific reports. The system has been proven to work, as long as you stick to it.

Secondly, it will encourage you to use a carefully chosen set of procedures, enabling you to tap mental powers and abilities which function very efficiently when you are undergoing a major lifestyle change. You may be amazed at how successful these procedures can be once you start to apply them systematically.

Thirdly, it is effective because it helps you to uncover the immediate triggers of your smoking and to eliminate your desire to smoke, along with the associated enjoyment and the satisfaction. Any method failing to address these motivating factors will fail to bring about a successful outcome.

Fourthly, the need for willpower is kept to the absolute minimum: it is unnecessary to fight a mental battle or make enormous efforts to change your behaviour. You do not need to feel any great stress or strain because you will not have to go to extreme lengths to stop smoking. Changing behaviour – learning new skills and unlearning old ones – can be done in a relaxed and natural way. Your brain will change its response to stimuli when the usual rewards are no longer present.

To obtain the best results, try to keep your mind as open as possible to the ideas in CBT. Free yourself from the worry that you have been unable to stop smoking in the past. The more you try to enjoy the process of participating in this CBT programme, the easier it should be to obtain the desired result. So try to have fun while you prove to yourself that you can give up smoking!

Noticing Your Automatic Smoking Chains

Every time you have a cigarette, an automatic chain of smoking responses is activated. In its most extreme form, this automatic chain can be carried out without a single conscious thought about what is happening.

A typical automatic chain consists of the following links:

1 Trigger stimulus.
2 Reach for packet.
3 Hold packet in one hand.
4 Remove one cigarette.
5 Place cigarette in mouth.
6 Find lighter or matches.
7 Light cigarette.
8 Inhale first puff.
9 Exhale first puff.
10 Place cigarette in ash tray.
11 Pick up cigarette from ash tray.
12 Inhale second puff.
13 Exhale second puff.
14 30 Another 9 or 30 puffs.
31 Put down cigarette.
32 Stub cigarette out.

This automatic chain, or a variation of it, is repeated every time a smoker has a cigarette. Because the chain is very difficult to stop once it has been started, you need to use a method to alert yourself when the chain is about to start. A simple technique has therefore been designed specifically for this purpose.

To help you notice each time you take a cigarette from the packet, place a rubber band around your packet. You will have to remove this before you take out each new cigarette. When you have finished taking out a cigarette (and completed the reduction card procedure described in the next section) make sure that your rubber band goes back onto your packet.

This rubber band serves two main purposes. Firstly. it is a protective device to give you an alarm signal every time you have a cigarette, to warn you that your automatic smoking chain is being "pulled' yet again. It therefore provides the first important step in successfully breaking the habit of smoking. By stopping the chain at the very beginning, you will eventually be able to gain control of the situation. Secondly, the rubber band will allow you to think about the trigger stimulus that is making you want to have a cigarette at the particular moment that you are removing it from the packet.

Using Your Daily Reduction Cards

It is important that you make a record of every cigarette you smoke from the date you start the CBT until you have completely stopped, so carry a pen or pencil with you at all times. Photocopy Appendix B, where you will find a set of Daily Reduction Cards for you to cut out of the photocopied sheet and insert into your cigarette pack. When you decide to have a cigarette, put a little '1' by the hour of day marked on the card. You will soon see what sort of smoking pattern emerges. Perhaps for you there are certain times of the day when you smoke more. These periods may be associated with tension or other moods or feelings.

Start a new card each day that you are in this Programme, and every night enter the total number of cigarettes you have smoked on your Progress Chart. You will be able to see the drop off in cigarette consumption with every day you use this Programme. Nine cards are provided, which will last until your D-Day (no later than Day 10). The Progress Chart shows a set of daily targets that you should aim to reach, starting with your current daily level as 100 per cent. These reduce by 50 to 60 per cent each day, which allows your smoking to gradually taper off.

If your current level is 20 cigarettes per day then you should aim to reduce this to 12 to 15 cigarettes on Day 1, 6 to 7 cigarettes on Day 2, 3 to 4 cigarettes on Day 3, 2 to 3 cigarettes on Day 4, 1 to 2 cigarettes on Day 5, and then 0 or 1 cigarette on Day 6. Your D-Day will be Day 7, when you definitely should not smoke.

If you are unable to keep to this decreasing series and have a 'hiccough' along the way, you will need to extend the series of preparation days – up to 9 days in total. I will describe the procedures for establishing the exact date for your D-Day in Chapter seven.

How to Deprogram Your Mind

At the moment, your brain contains the mental programming of a smoker, and your biocomputer automatically plays the programs that give you the desire to smoke when it is presented with certain kinds of stimulation. When you see, hear, smell or feel a trigger stimulus – or if you have not smoked for a certain period of time, and the nicotine level in your body is running low – a message is automatically sent to the biocomputer, asking you to top up your nicotine levels. The biocomputer responds and begins to correct the situation. In order to top up the amount of nicotine in the body, you must be made to want to smoke a cigarette. The biocomputer sends a craving feeling to your conscious mind, and you then experience a conscious desire for a cigarette. Quite automatically, you pick up a cigarette and smoke it to satisfy your craving, and the brain gives you a conscious feeling of pleasure or satisfaction in its place. This cycle of events is repeated over and over again.

The cycle looks like this:

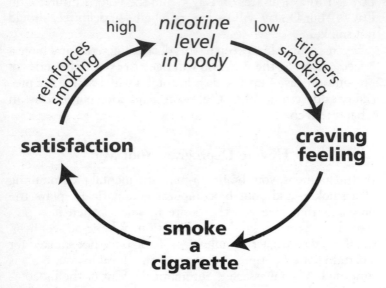

In this case, your smoking is strongly rewarded. Notice also that the sequence switches from conscious experience **(in bold)** to unconscious programming (*in italics*) quite automatically. This makes it very difficult to intervene and interrupt the cycle.

It is important to remember that your biocomputer did not always operate in this way. Once upon a time you would never have craved a cigarette. It should not be long before you return to that state. All you need to do is to change your current programming. In effect, your mind and body will revert back to their original state before you took up smoking. All the learning that took place during your initiation to smoking, and after your habit was established, will be completely reversed. For example, once upon a time you enjoyed a meal or a drink without needing to have a smoke. Perhaps these days you always smoke after your dinner and while having a cup of tea or coffee. The signal comes – 'dinner over, coffee made' – and the biocomputer automatically responds by playing the 'I want a cigarette now' program. You respond automatically and, if possible, light up.

Because of the multiple repetitions of the pairing of coffee with smoking, you now respond automatically to pro-grammed instructions to smoke and this makes you feel as though you have very little choice. If you decide not to have a cigarette, you become involved in an extremely difficult battle. You are forced to use your willpower to resist the temptation of having a cigarette. If you rely on your willpower, you are likely to lose, and you may have to suffer the consequences of withdrawal. The sequence then looks like this:

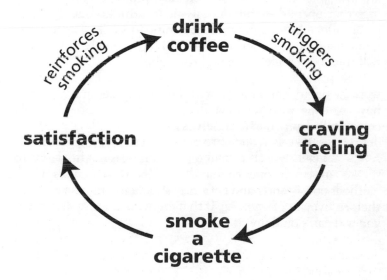

In this case, by not smoking you are in effect punishing your-self, and you are likely to give into your craving when it becomes stronger. Once again, the sequence of events switches from conscious to unconscious, which means that you have great difficulty controlling it. While you may feel pleased with yourself at an intellectual level for resisting the drive to smoke, your act of consciously resisting smoking is not being rewarded at a feeling level. It is the feeling level that dominates the experience of the addict. This is why willpower is not enough. You are placing your feelings in conflict with your thoughts. CBT will enable you to remove the inconsistency by changing your experience of smoking from a pleasant to an unpleasant experience and eliminating your desire to smoke altogether.

When we talk about giving up smoking, or eliminating dependency on the drug nicotine, we are talking about deprogramming that part of your mind that makes you restless and unhappy when you deny yourself a cigarette. This is the radical difference between using CBT and many other methods that are available. CBT uses psychological principles and procedures that operate simultaneously at the thinking and feeling levels. Once the feeling that you want to smoke is gone, the immediate cause of your smoking will have been removed. You will then be completely free of the habit.

It is entirely up to you how thoroughly you are prepared to work at deprogramming your desire to smoke, and thus not have to cope with that awful craving feeling. Some people completely deprogram themselves in a matter of days, and their desire to smoke is reduced to zero. Others deprogram themselves sufficiently well to make the fight against the desire to smoke an easier one to handle. Nobody who uses these methods consistently and patiently should fail to destroy all of their enjoyment of smoking. If that enjoyment is not destroyed, you will carry on doing it.

Program 1

When you draw on a cigarette, allowing hot, poisonous fumes to enter your respiratory system and burn your throat, irritate and destroy the delicate tissues in your lungs, and eventually cause a 'smoker's cough', how is it possible that you can feel pleasure, enjoyment, and satisfaction?

The answer, of course, is that your brain naturally gives you a feeling of pleasure when nicotine enters your body and dopamine is released in the pleasure centres. At the same time, your body has adapted to the naturally unpleasant sensations of the smoke and is now fully capable of screening most of them out.

Consider what happens to non-smokers, when for some reason they decide to smoke a cigarette. With the first puff the heart begins to beat more rapidly, mainly due to the effect of the drug nicotine. The amount of oxygen absorbed into the bloodstream decreases because the poisonous gas carbon monoxide is absorbed instead. With a lowered supply of oxygen to the brain, the person will probably begin to feel dizzy and their head will start to ache. They may feel quite ill and experience nausea. If they try to smoke more than one cigarette, they may even vomit.

How does a smoker's programming become so powerful? There are many different ways. Among the most important are social pressure, cigarette advertising and social conditioning. Rebelling against authority figures is also a factor, especially in the 10- to 14-year-old age group, when most smokers take up the habit. Once smoking has started, all of these pressures are reinforced by the addictive qualities of the drug nicotine, and Pro-Cigarette Programs (PCPs) become deeply embedded in the mind.

Here is an example of the kind of program that automatically begins to run through your mind when you light a cigarette:

Ah . . . that feels better. I really needed this cigarette. I'm enjoying this cigarette. It satisfies me. It relaxes me. I feel more alive, more stimulated. I am enjoying myself. That's better. I feel good.

The aim of using CBT is to completely remove this deluding programming, so that when you inhale the poisonous fumes of a cigarette, your biocomputer does not play you this misleading message. When you draw cigarette smoke into your lungs, you need to be told what is really happening to your body. This can be achieved by deliberately and consciously repeating a more accurate program in your mind during the process of smoking. Your new program must state exactly what messages you want your biocomputer to produce in the future. At first you will still be under the influence of your old programming, and you won't experience all the effects of the new program immediately. But, by repeating the new program with each and every cigarette, your biocomputer will gradually absorb it and repeat it during the act of smoking. Your biocomputer, like any computer, will not object to the new program if it is consistent.

A highly effective substitute program is given below. I call it Program 1. Please learn it and repeat it to yourself every time you smoke a cigarette from now on. When you do so regularly you will quickly discover that your cigarette consumption is dropping rather dramatically. Within 24 hours your consumption should be reduced by 25 to 50 per cent. It is necessary to learn it by heart and use it every time you have a cigarette from now on.

PROGRAM 1

As I smoke I realize that:
This cigarette is giving me <u>n</u>o satisfaction.   **N**
This is an <u>u</u>npleasant experience.   **U**
This cigarette is making me feel <u>r</u>otten.   **R**
I am losing the <u>d</u>esire to smoke.   **D**

The following condensed version may be help you to memorize Program 1:

<u>N</u>O SATISFACTION   **N**
<u>U</u>NPLEASANT   **U**
<u>R</u>OTTEN   **R**
<u>D</u>ESIRE   **D**

The 4 key letters N, U, R, D spell a made-up word or mnemonic 'NURD' (similar to the word 'NERD') to help you to remember the whole program.

Notice that NURD operates at the thinking, feeling and behavioural levels at the same time. NURD tells your biocomputer that you are not enjoying smoking any more and that it is giving you no satisfaction – and it does this while you are in the act of smoking. In other words, the goal to overcome smoking is being realized at all three levels at the same time. The levels are no longer in conflict. This is more consistent than willpower, which always generates conflict.

From now on, you should smoke every cigarette deliberately and with concentration. If you are able to, stop whatever you are doing for a few minutes and really concentrate on your smoking. Repeat the program to yourself. When you say to yourself, 'This is an unpleasant experience,' think about the parts of our body which are directly affected by this unpleasant experience – your tongue, mouth, throat and lungs; and feel especially the extra strain being placed upon your heart. At first you may not actually experience anything as being very unpleasant. However, keep repeating the program every time you smoke. Within a day, you will notice that this has dramatically affected the way you experience cigarette smoking.

It is important that you use Program 1 every time you have a cigarette. Recite it automatically to yourself while you are smoking.

Remember to make use of the letters NURD that are printed at the top of the Daily Reduction Cards. Use each letter as you glance at the card in the packet, to remind you of Program 1 while you are smoking:

N = No satisfaction U = Unpleasant R = Rotten D = Desire

Think or say a line of Program 1 to yourself with each new puff of your cigarette. Smoke the cigarette right through and then stub it out. Make sure you've marked your Daily Reduction

Card in the correct time slot, put it safely back inside your cigarette packet, and replace the rubber band around the packet. Everything is now in place for your next cigarette.

Why Program 1 Is More Effective Than Using Willpower

We have already illustrated one way in which CBT is superior to willpower. The feeling, thinking and behavioural levels are brought into line. Here, we look at another aspect of the problem with willpower as a means for changing your behaviour.

It is a basic principle of CBT not to use willpower. Why? Let's look at the consequences of using willpower. As a smoker, there are two conflicting parts to your personality. For convenience we shall label these 'Smoker' and 'Non-smoker'. Smoker is the dependent, emotional, more childish part of your character who tends to give in easily to problems and stress, and who usually ends up craving a smoke. Non-smoker is the more independent, rational, and mature adult who really does want to give up smoking and develop more healthy ways of coping with difficulties.

Let's look at what happens when you try to use willpower to stop smoking when you have this kind of 'double personality'. Consider two groups of smokers. The first group are trying to give up by themselves using their willpower. They haven't smoked for half an hour and are beginning to experience the desire to smoke. The Non-smoker part of their personality decides to put it off and not have a cigarette for a while. They carry on with some activity but, all the time, Smoker is generating thoughts about smoking and the desire to smoke actually becomes stronger. The more Non-smoker resists having a cigarette, the more Smoker feels like smoking, and the stronger the person's conscious desire actually becomes. There is now a complete split in their personality, and they feel torn between smoking and non-smoking. Finally, there is a complete breakdown, and the desire to smoke becomes so strong that Smoker wins. They light up, and exactly as expected, enjoy it. The desire to smoke will return in another half an hour and the whole cycle of events will be repeated.

What does this do to the programming inside the head? It reinforces smoking very strongly! When feelings of tension are reduced immediately after a cigarette is lit, the act of smoking is strongly rewarded. By using willpower to stop smoking, the desire to smoke becomes stronger and the smoking habit is unlikely to be changed. When the desire to smoke is at its strongest, the smoker is rewarded by the enjoyment of the cigarette. Thus, using willpower makes it more difficult to eliminate smoking, because the mental programs which cause the smoking become even more deeply reinforced.

Now let's look at a group of smokers who are using Program 1. When smokers in this group begin to experience the desire to smoke, instead of delaying lighting up and letting the desire get stronger, they tackle the problem while it is still weak. These smokers sit down and, while lighting up, begin to control what they are thinking about. They think and say to themselves the four lines of NURD. They begin to repeat, 'This cigarette is giving me no satisfaction,' and they take a deep inhalation from the cigarette, deliberately making themselves aware of the unpleasant effects that the smoke is having. This is relatively easy to do because the desire to smoke is not all that strong. Then, consciously saying to themselves, 'This is an unpleasant experience', the smokers take another deep inhalation. Again, with one deep inhalation each time, the lines 'This cigarette is making me feel rotten' and 'I am losing the desire to smoke' are repeated.

By this stage, the smoking experience is becoming uncomfortable and unpleasant. The biocomputer begins to interpret what is happening to the smoker's body more accurately. Smokers using this procedure actually do begin to experience smoking as an unpleasant and sometimes even a painful experience. Smokers in this group finish their cigarettes to the very end, and, realizing that it is extremely uncomfortable to smoke in this manner, deliberately use the cigarette itself to begin the important task of destroying the programs that are responsible for keeping the habit going. Once they've put the cigarette out, it may be several hours before they experience the desire to smoke again.

There will be variation between individuals but, for each person using Program 1, the time between cigarettes will increase and the desire decrease until it completely fades away. Compare that with smokers using willpower, whose craving gets stronger the longer they delay having another cigarette.

Advantages of Using Program 1

1 Program 1 is most effective when the desire to smoke is still weak. By smoking when you feel like having a cigarette, and using Program 1, you are extinguishing the learned association between the trigger and the reward.
2 By using willpower and delaying lighting up, smokers will inevitably break down and reward themselves by smoking. Rewarding the behaviour makes it stronger and also strengthens the desire.
3 By lighting up while the desire is still relatively weak, the smoker can use Program 1 effectively. By controlling what they are thinking about, and taking a deep inhalation of smoke, the biocomputer learns the true consequences of smoking. This makes smoking unpleasant when the desire is weak, and eventually makes the desire fade away completely.
4 By using Program 1 effectively, a smoker will spend the next few hours in a comparatively calm state. With willpower only, the smoker will spend the next hour thinking about smoking in a state of moderate tension.

The more effectively you use Program 1, the less often you will feel like smoking and the sooner you will quit smoking altogether.

James' Progress

The techniques of this chapter can be illustrated by the experiences of James. On Tuesday, James felt that he couldn't stop smoking in the company of other smokers, as he would feel anti-social. The belief that not smoking in front of other smokers is anti-social was explored. It was pointed out to James that he should be aware of thoughts related to feeling anti-social amongst smokers. If he noticed such a thought, he was told to say to himself, 'Just because I'm with other smokers, it does not mean I need to smoke. Stopping smoking is not anti-social.' All the CBT techniques were explained to James, and he felt confident that he could apply all of them. He liked the idea of learning to become a non-smoker and saw it as a challenge. He also felt that a gradual reduction of cigarettes was more realistic.

James felt excited about starting his new challenge. On day one, he put the rubber band on his cigarette packet, inserted the reduction card and started to take note of his triggers to smoke. James felt that he knew all of his triggers. However, he was surprised that, every time he smoked, it was related to a trigger, and he discovered many new ones.

Summary

- Keep a rubber band on your cigarette packet so that you are unable to smoke automatically.
- Learn Program 1 (NURD) and automatically say it to yourself every time you smoke.
- Make a note of every cigarette you smoke on your Daily Reduction Cards from now on. At the end of each day enter your total consumption on your Progress Chart.

Day 2: Wednesday – Regaining Control from Automatic Pilot

One of the most important functions of the brain is to control essential life processes such as our breathing, blood supply, and digestive processes. The brain and nervous system, together with the endocrine and immune systems, keep us ticking over, whatever we are doing, and also when we are sleeping or unconscious. The brain enables us to perceive the environment, to learn and use language, to learn new skills, to imagine and create new things, and to remember and understand our experiences.

The brain and nervous system are therefore able to control things that are pre-programmed and to automatically perform all of those functions that keep us alive. Then other functions, which are 'optional extras', are added to the main bodily functions through the process of learning. This is where many of our problems begin.

Our physical and biological make-up has evolved over a couple of million years. We are built to live as hunter-gatherers but live as sedentary consumers. Our physical environment consists of the atmosphere, the land, and the water from which we draw sustenance. Unfortunately, much of our environment is now polluted with all kinds of unfriendly chemicals.

Our social environment consists of family, friends, neighbours, work colleagues and many other people with whom we have relationships. This has both emotionally supportive and less supportive elements. Contemporary urban living includes a diverse collection of hazardous activities and habits associated with our so-called 'progressive' lifestyle. One of these is nicotine addiction, in which toxic fumes and chemicals are inhaled into our bodies as tobacco smoke.

Smoking has been represented by the tobacco industry as a 'cool' thing to do. For many generations of men, and for the current generation of women, smoking has been a rite of passage into adulthood, but it is a habit that they have inevitably regretted when they are older. At first, the smoker has to put some effort into learning how to smoke a cigarette, inhale the smoke without coughing, and look as if it is enjoyable at the same time. In reality, while the young smoker may put on a front of trying to look 'cool', few people enjoy smoking on the first occasion of doing so. On the contrary, it is a highly unpleasant experience. Eventually, however, the smoker adapts to all of the unpleasant bodily sensations, a physical dependency on nicotine and a psychological dependency on the ritual develop, and smoking automatically occurs whenever there is a desire to do so. That is how the smoking habit is acquired.

Pro-Cigarette Programs (PCPs)

While this analysis provides a general description of how people acquire habits and skills, there are large individual differences in the way people learn to cope with events. On seeing a dog in the park, one person may go up to it and pat it (and feel safe and secure), while another person may try to avoid the dog (because they feel frightened or insecure near dogs). The first person is programmed to react positively towards dogs because their experience with dogs suggests there is nothing to be frightened about, while the second person is programmed to react negatively towards dogs, perhaps because of an earlier frightening experience.

In similar fashion, as a smoker, you have been programmed to react positively towards cigarettes and the inhalation of cigarette smoke. In fact, you have many programs in your biocomputer that are specifically designed to keep you smoking. Your primary task over the next few days is to discover as many of these Pro-Cigarette Programs (PCPs) as possible. Then you will replace them with programs that are beneficial to you.

Impossible? Not at all.

The PCPs which encourage you smoke have been drummed into your brain by a large number of forces, most of which were external. Some of the main ones are:

- When you were in your teens, a desire to rebel against people who have tried to control your behaviour – parents, teachers, and other authority figures.
- The addictive properties of nicotine.
- Cigarette advertising making cigarette smoking appear cool.
- Peer pressure from smokers among your family, or friends or other people you want to identify with.
- The idea that smoking helps you control your weight.

The addictive properties of nicotine become more powerful, the more that you smoke. As we saw in Chapter three, every time your nicotine level runs low, and you top it up again by having a quick fix, smoking behaviour is strongly reinforced. Your smoking behaviour, including your desire to smoke, becomes linked to a whole host of stimuli in your immediate surroundings that act as triggers for your smoking. Whenever a trigger is present, your desire to have a cigarette increases. These associations have become deeply embedded in your mind by frequent repetition and reward. Every time you smoke a cigarette, your pleasure centres in your brain receive a shot of dopamine that reinforces a link between the desire to smoke, the sensations of smoking, and aspects of your external environment. Eventually, those features of the situation which are repeatedly associated with smoking will become triggers which set off your desire to smoke. Triggers and PCPs have become a routine part of your life. For most of the time, you have been blissfully unaware that they are controlling your behaviour. They operate as automatically as your breathing, sitting in a chair, or walking. They just happen.

How A PCP Operates

Imagine the following scenario. You and some other smokers are watching television. One of the TV characters lights a cigarette. What happens in the room several moments after that? It is very likely that all the smokers will have reached for their cigarettes and will now have a cigarette burning. In spite of the regularity and uniformity of their actions, it is unlikely that they will be aware of what made them all have a cigarette at that particular point in time. In fact, it is a hidden program in each of their minds that has made them feel like smoking a cigarette whenever they observe someone else light up. If you ask any of the smokers why they lit up at that moment, the probable answer would be, 'I just felt like it.'

Here is what actually happened to the smokers:

Pro-Cigarette Program– Whenever anyone lights a cigarette, I will automatically feel like smoking.

Trigger – Someone on television lights a cigarette.

Automatic Response – I feel like smoking a cigarette.

As a smoker, you are programmed to respond automatically to many different trigger situations. You have almost no control over these automatic responses. Just as you are programmed to feel frightened when threatened with danger, you are programmed to feel like having a cigarette when presented with a situation which is associated with smoking in your mind.

Here is another example:

Pro-Cigarette Program – Whenever you feel upset with someone, you will automatically feel like smoking.

Trigger – Husband/wife/partner comes home late from work and the dinner is spoiled in the oven.

Automatic Response – You feel like smoking.

Each and every PCP needs to be individually deprogrammed so that in the future, when these situations occur, you will not automatically respond by smoking a cigarette. You need a technique for discovering all of your trigger situations. Then, when you have identified each of them, you need a technique for responding differently. The process of discovering trigger situations will be helped by Program 2.

Program 2

Program 2 will make you aware of your smoking triggers. It is essential to have it firmly embedded in your mind. With a little bit of practice, every time you smoke you should be able to discover precisely what it was that triggered off the feeling. The whole process can be remembered as 'WEST-D'.

PROGRAM 2	
What is the trigger?	**W**
Each time I feel like smoking	**E**
Stop	**S**
Think	**T**
Deprogram	**D**

So, every time you feel like smoking a cigarette, you should follow Program 2 (WEST- D). Every time you feel like having a cigarette, you must recognize that one of your PCPs has been activated by a trigger. You must search for that trigger so that you can learn to deprogram yourself. Once you have discovered what it was that triggered off the desire to smoke, you have a golden opportunity to deprogram the automatic response so that, the next time the situation occurs, you will be less likely to automatically light up. Methods of deprogramming are described later in this chapter.

You may have to go through the deprogramming process several times to get rid of each trigger. How often you need to deprogram will depend on how deeply embedded each program is, and on how forcefully you deprogram it. However, in a very short time, you will find yourself thinking, 'Whenever that used to happen, I felt like a cigarette. Now, I never smoke in that situation!' The realization that you have changed your habits so easily is quite astonishing.

You probably have dozens of triggers, but all of the common ones are going to occur over the next few days. As and when they occur, you should deprogram them. Then light up, have a cigarette, and say Program 1.

A few triggers occur only on rare occasions, and they may not appear during the next few days. However, by the time one of them does appear, your general resistance to smoking will be a lot stronger and you will be able to cope with the trigger and not smoke.

On D-Day and afterwards, there will still be times when an old program is triggered, giving you the desire to smoke. Its effect may only last for a very short period, sometimes as short as a few seconds; but, even then, go through the same deprogramming process that you will learn in the next section. Make sure that, the next time the situation occurs, you won't feel like smoking. Remember that your mind is a biocomputer and, like an electronic computer, it has no will of its own. It is not fussy about what is programmed into it. It is as comfortable containing Anti-Cigarette Programs (ACPs) in its memory files as it is containing Pro-Cigarette Programs. To quit smoking for life, you should repeatedly deprogram your automatic responses every time you feel like smoking. Every time you feel that you want to have a cigarette, that is a signal for you to use Program 2.

Triggers

We are all programmed in our own individual ways, and we all respond differently according to the individual events in our lives. However, we can all deprogram our automatic responses in the same way. Here is a list of some of the more common triggers:

- waking up in the morning
- finishing lunch or dinner
- finishing washing the dishes
- sitting down in a chair to relax
- turning on the TV
- drinking a cup of tea or coffee, or some alcohol
- being in a bar
- feeling in a bad mood
- feeling rejected or lonely
- being with friends or people you like/don't like
- being offered a cigarette by another smoker
- seeing someone else light up
- seeing a cigarette advertisement
- seeing cigarettes on sale
- starting your car
- answering the telephone
- starting/finishing something
- preparing to go to bed

Using Program 2, you will become very aware of which particular things trigger off your desire to smoke. As soon as you realize what it is that is triggering the response to smoke, deprogram it! Keep a record of the triggers you have discovered on your Personal Trigger List. Update this list at regular intervals as you discover more triggers, and one by one you will be able to eliminate them.

Personal Trigger List

1 _____

2 _____

3 _____

4 _____

5 _____

6 _____

7 _____

8 _____

9 _____

10 _____

11 _____

12 _____

13 _____

14 _____

15 _____

16 _____

17 _____

18 _____

19 _____

20 _____

21 _____

22 _____

23 _____

24 _____

Deprogramming With Words

There are two methods for changing your automatic programs:

1 Deprogramming by using *Verbal Commands*.
2 Reprogramming by using *Imagery Rehearsal*.

There are two major ways you can feed new information into your biocomputer: through words and through images. Your biocomputer is open to both channels of information. Before you can use images to reprogram new behaviour, you must first use words to deprogram the behaviour you no longer want. You can start using verbal commands for deprogramming right away. Reprogramming with images should be started tomorrow and is described in the next chapter.

Employ deprogramming as soon as you become aware that you are feeling like having a cigarette. Here's an example: imagine that you have just sat down in front of the television. You pick up your cigarettes. Reaching for the cigarettes is a signal for you to think of Program 2. You must go through the following **WEST-D** routine : **W – WHAT** is the trigger? **E – EACH** time I feel like smoking I must **S – STOP**. I **T– THINK** to myself: 'I feel like a smoke now. What is triggering that feeling?' Then you discover that it was because you had just turned on the TV and had sat down to watch a film. You realize that you always light up after you have switched on the TV and sat down. It seems perfectly natural to reach for the cigarette packet in this situation.

Now that you have discovered what it was that triggered the desire to smoke, you should begin to **D – DEPROGRAM** it while you are still aware of it, so that it will not make you feel like smoking the next time you turn the TV on. To remove the programs that cause you to smoke, you need to feed completely new instructions into the biocomputer. These new instructions must be specific, clear and to the point.

66

These verbal commands to your biocomputer will deprogram the desire to smoke if you use them repeatedly and in an assertive, demanding and forcible manner. You must say the command as though you really mean it! By repeating the new instructions forcibly, you are giving your biocomputer no option but to accept them. Be very clear about what you are trying to achieve. You are not trying to build up your willpower. You are ordering your biocomputer to stop producing the automatic response 'I feel like a cigarette'.

Here is an example of how to carry out deprogramming. Imagine that you are having a cup of coffee. You feel like smoking a cigarette and use Program 2. You identify **What is the trigger?** You **Stop, Think, and Deprogram**. The last three steps are crucial. Here are some specific instructions that you could feed into your biocomputer:

Wanting a cigarette now is just an automatic response to having a cup of coffee.
Just because I am having a cup of coffee, it doesn't mean I have to feel like smoking. The next time I have a cup of coffee, I refuse to automatically feel like smoking.
Whenever I sit down to drink coffee. I won't automatically think of having a cigarette. I won't be made to smoke just because I'm having a cup of coffee.

Your own verbal commands can of course say exactly what you want them to say. Be specific. Be emphatic. Be demanding. The language may sometimes be unprintable!

As soon as you feel like smoking a cigarette, you should go through the three main steps:

1 STOP (S)
Don't light up yet. Think of Program 2.

2 THINK (T)
Be aware that you are responding automatically. Ask yourself, 'What am I responding to?' When you discover what it is:

3 DEPROGRAM (D)

Begin to talk to your biocomputer in a firm and demanding manner. Repeat the instructions over and over again to make a very strong impression on your biocomputer. Your biocomputer will accept anything you program into it if you constantly and firmly repeat the idea you want it to accept.

This process needn't take up a lot of time. A few minutes spent repeating these ideas in your mind will pay dividends. By the very next day, you can expect to notice a situation when you would once have smoked, but this time you do not automatically reach for a cigarette. When you realize that this process is actually working, and that your behaviour is changing quite dramatically, you will experience a great deal of satisfaction and enjoyment.

When you have gone through the Three Steps of the WEST-D sequence and have told yourself not to respond by wanting a cigarette the next time, carry on with what you started to do. Drink a cup of coffee, begin watching television, or whatever it was, while having a cigarette. It is vital that you smoke this time because you do actually feel like a smoke. But remember to say Program 1. The whole purpose of this procedure is to deprogram the automatic responses so that the feeling or desire to smoke stops coming automatically as a response to what you are doing. So have the cigarette, but only after you have used the three steps and forcibly told yourself not to respond automatically next time.

As you continue to use Program 2 and the three steps, you will notice that you have lost the desire to smoke in each particular trigger situation. Smoke a cigarette afterwards (if you still feel like one) and use Program 1. Finally, don't forget to mark it on your Daily Reduction Card.

Why Must New Programs Be Repeated So Mechanically?

Memorizing them and repeating them helps you to implant them deeply into your mind. Just reading them will not allow you to use them as active and effective tools to rid you completely of the need to inhale poisonous tobacco smoke. Try to memorize Programs 1 and 2 and use them from now on whenever you feel like a cigarette. You will find that, by putting some effort into memorizing them, you can deeply embed them in your mind, and they will soon function as automatically as the programs which keep you smoking. If they are well learned, they will simply flash into your mind whenever you need them and you won't need to make any great effort to use them.

It is an extremely valuable exercise to list all the verbal commands that you discover. Typical examples might be:

The next time I wake up in the morning I will not automatically feel like lighting a cigarette. The next time I have a cup of coffee I will not automatically feel like having a smoke.' *The next time I put the washing in the washing machine I will not automatically feel like a smoke.*

Most smokers have between 25 and 30 different triggers. If you reinforce the deprogramming process by writing down each verbal command, you will be able to read them through in the evening and have material you can use to begin reprogramming yourself with new desirable behaviour. As you continue to use these programs, you will notice that your daily consumption of cigarettes will continue to fall without a great effort.

James' Progress

James noticed many new triggers and used Programs 1 and 2 very consistently. He saw the whole experience as an interesting and enjoyable journey of discovery. By the end of Day 2, he had reduced his consumption to 10 cigarettes.

His satisfaction and enjoyment with smoking had significantly reduced. He kept going, even though his confidence waned at times. Knowing that the progress so far was quite good, he kept a daily record of his progress on his chart and hung it over his computer at work. His work colleagues gave him their support – even the other smokers. This was a great help to him. He looked forward to the weekend and to the idea that he would set a D-Day in the near future.

Summary

- Use Program 1 every time you smoke.
- Use Program 2 every time you feel like smoking.
- Deprogram yourself using the three steps. Every time you feel like a smoke, remember to STOP, THINK (What is the trigger?), and DEPROGRAM with strong verbal commands ('The next time I . . . , I will refuse to smoke. Don't send me that smoking feeling. I'll smoke when I choose to do so.').
- Keep a list of your triggers.
- Make a list of your personal verbal commands.
- Keep a rubber band on your packet at all times.
- Complete your Daily Reduction Card and, at the end of the day, record the day's total on your Progress Chart.

Day 3: Thursday – Calming Your Restless Mind

As a smoker, you will probably agree that smoking often makes you feel calmer or relaxed. 'Feeling calmer' is one of the most commonly reported subjective effects of smoking. Typically, smokers report feeling calmer while smoking. Smoking may help you to feel more at ease when you feel nervous or embarrassed. The ability to relax is seen as being one of the main benefits of smoking and many smokers smoke more when they are worried or 'stressed out'. Being able to relax provides a justification for continuing the habit.

You will learn how to make use of two of your natural abilities to make a breakthrough as a calm, happy and successful non-smoker. These abilities are your powers of *imagination* and *relaxation*. Both of these abilities are universal, even among people who claim not to have them. Some people say they cannot image things in their imagination for example. However, research in psychophysiology has shown that everybody dreams every time they have a night's sleep. When we dream, we are using our creative imagination. Dream images generate alternative possibilities to those of everyday, waking reality. So, if you can dream, you can also learn to generate images while you are awake. When you are daydreaming about something, and your mind wanders away from some mundane task to something more pleasant, your mental imagery is fired into action. Why not learn to use your imaging ability to achieve something really healthy and useful, such as giving up smoking?

As you learn to use your creative imagination, you will discover that your ability to form vivid images depends upon your mental state. If you are feeling tense or upset, you may not be able to produce the images that you want, or they may be very fleeting or poorly controlled. However, mental imagery becomes more vivid and easier to control when you are relaxed.

Imagery Rehearsal

This section will guide you to use your powers of imagination to quit smoking. You will know from everyday experience that you can imagine future events and plan how to deal with them before they actually happen. On some occasions, these visualizations may be rather pessimistic and you will tend to imagine things going wrong. On other occasions, the images are optimistic and you will see how things could work out if things go well. Now that you have decided to give up smoking, please use your images positively – that is, use your ability to rehearse situations where you will cope happily in the future, without having a cigarette.

The imagery method is very powerful indeed. Scientific trials have shown that the use of mental imagery to rehearse future performance helps golfers, athletes, and orchestra conductors to improve their skill. Patients have also been helped to cope with, and recover more quickly from, operations. You can learn to use these same mental processes to achieve your goal of becoming a successful non-smoker.

Everything that you imagine will be processed at different levels of consciousness. One of the key features of your images is their meaning. Your images will suggest new programs for your biocomputer that will influence your future thoughts, feelings, and actions. A person's belief in what she or he can achieve is a powerful determinant of what they actually do achieve. Thus your images of yourself, of what you can and can't do, and how you will feel as a result, all help to determine the outcome of your desire to stop smoking. Rehearsing images of yourself not smoking, and seeing yourself coping well with the more difficult triggers, will help these things to happen.

In order to actually become a beautifully balanced, calm and collected non-smoker, you must firstly be able to see this new you in your imagination. Try it now. Close your eyes and enter your private world of imagination. It is here that you make the decisions about the kind of person you would like to be and what you would most like to achieve. Try to see yourself as a happy and successful non-smoker.

Mentally rehearse a situation in which you would normally smoke a cigarette but see yourself coping without that cigarette. See yourself coping successfully, remaining perfectly happy and at ease without a cigarette. See it really happening: imagine as vividly as possible who else is there, what they are doing, how you are feeling, and how good it is not to be smoking in that particular situation.

The more you practise trigger situations in your imagination, especially while you are in a relaxed frame of mind, the more confidently you will be able to deal with these situations in real life. Eventually, all of your triggers can be completely eliminated.

Let's look at this process in more detail. Having started to deprogram your old smoking behaviour, your biocomputer now has the capacity for some new programs and so you can reprogram new, non-smoking behaviour. PCPs can be replaced by ACPs, and imagery rehearsal is one of the most effective ways of doing this. Your experience with Program 2 should have provided you with useful information about some of your principal triggers.

Some triggers should now be losing their power as a result of using Program 2. You may even have had a cup of tea or coffee without having an accompanying smoke, perhaps for the first time in many years! Others may be more resistant and require more repetition to be removed completely. Imagery rehearsal provides a useful method for building new behaviours and feelings to fill the gap left by smoking.

Make a list of triggers as they occur during the day, or write out a list in the evening. Use your Daily Record Card to remind you exactly when you did smoke.

Imagery Exercise

Allow about five minutes for this exercise. Sit in a comfortable chair, away from the TV and other distractions. Try to become as relaxed as possible. You may even decide to try this last thing at night, before you go to sleep.

As you relax, think of one of your triggers. With your eyes closed, replay that particular scene as vividly as possible. But, this time, imagine that you didn't actually smoke at all. Mentally practise the situation as you would really like it to have been. Imagine it as vividly as possible, pretending that you didn't have a smoke. Repeat the image a few times, remaining as calm and relaxed as possible. When you can achieve a clear and vivid image of yourself coping calmly with the trigger but without smoking, you know that you will be better able to cope with that trigger in real life.

You should practise imagery rehearsal at least once each day for a few minutes to eliminate every trigger, one by one.

Calming Your Mind

We know that many people continue to smoke, despite being well aware that smoking is a lethal and unnatural activity. Why?

It is very common for people to become so concerned about their health that they try to give up smoking. Many do so. Many try and don't succeed. Some give up for an hour, a day, a few weeks, a few months, even a few years. But why do people start smoking again?

While you are in the process of deprogramming your old PCPs, and replacing them with behaviour that is free from the need to smoke, your consumption of cigarettes begins to drop. This causes a problem, which often defeats many would-be non-smokers. The problem has two parts:

1 Physically, you are addicted to nicotine;
2 Mentally, automatic programs are triggering a desire to smoke.

The Physical Addiction

The addiction is easy to understand. Because you are smoking less, your body begins to react and demands its regular fix of nicotine. Because you don't feel like smoking so often, your body and brain become desperate to get a supply of the drug nicotine. Your body will begin to put pressure on you to smoke, in order to satisfy your addiction to nicotine. As you continue to deny your body the amount of nicotine that it is used to, your body responds by craving it, giving you pangs of urging, and tensing up. The more you deny your body its fix, the more tense and stressed you will become. Having a cigarette will temporarily relieve the tension by satisfying the addiction. However, reducing your nicotine level tends to make you irritable and uncomfortable, and it is at this stage that many smokers who are trying to stop smoking give in, rather than carrying on feeling so tense and miserable.

However, the tension in your body can be relieved in a far more satisfying and natural way than by smoking – by learning to relax. Instead of holding on to the tension that is building up in your body, you can learn how to let it go by learning to relax deeply. It is very simple to let tension flow out of the body, but most people carry tension around with them all day and, even at night, as they fall asleep, their fists are clenched and their muscles are tight. So many people suffer from headaches, ulcers, general irritability and nervousness, simply because they do not know how to relieve themselves of the everyday stresses and tensions built up in the body.

One of the most effective ways of releasing tension is by using meditation. This is a way of relaxing your mind and body very deeply and, by using this technique, you can reduce the desire to smoke by relieving the body of the tension that tends to build up when deprived of nicotine. A method of meditation is described in the next section of this book (see page 81).

The Mental Process

As you smoke less and less, the PCPs in your biocomputer will be played over and over to tempt you to smoke. They do this in an extremely seductive and subtle way. Your mind generates and invents the most amazingly convincing reasons why you should have a smoke. These reasons are often so cleverly thought up that, if you are not aware of what is happening, you will accept them and quite happily have a cigarette. The addicted and deprived part of the brain is trying to trick the rational part by using *rationalizations*. These are illusory or delusory reasons to smoke.

In reality there are absolutely no good reasons to smoke, but your mind is so subtle and creative that it is trying to hoodwink the sensible part that wants to quit smoking. Unless you become fully aware of what is happening, these rationalizations will enter the mind quietly, and sit there until you have got used to them being there. When you have almost automatically accepted one of them as true, you go and light up quite spontaneously. Clearly, you need a way of dealing with this.

Here is a typical example.

Let's assume that you have not smoked for the past two hours or so, and you are sitting down with a cup of coffee. You realize that because you have been deprogramming yourself so well over the last couple of days, you didn't even feel like smoking when you sat down with your cup of coffee. You are quite enjoying the fact that you are having a cup of coffee and not even feeling like smoking. You have been giving verbal commands to your biocomputer not to send you the desire to smoke when you have a cup of coffee, and you have reinforced this by using imagery rehearsal in the evening to practise having a cup and enjoying it without smoking.

Now you pick up an old magazine and, as you turn the pages

you spot an attractive cigarette advertisement. There is a picture of your favourite brand of cigarettes. Immediately another of your PCPs begins to play. You now feel like smoking.

You think immediately of Program 2 and the three steps. You say to yourself: 'STOP. This is an opportunity to get rid of another trigger. THINK. What am I responding to? Obviously it's the advertisement. START DEPROGRAMMING. I refuse to obey that program. The next time I see an attractive cigarette advertisement, I will not automatically feel like a cigarette. I absolutely refuse to be forced to smoke every time I see a cigarette ad. I don't want to be a robot. I don't want to react mechanically. I don't want to be forced to smoke just because I see a cigarette advertisement.'

Having finished giving your biocomputer these stern verbal commands, you carry on reading your magazine. But, of course, the desire to smoke is still in you, and you are still thinking about smoking. Your mind seems obsessed with thoughts about smoking, and how much you would like to have a cigarette right now. Perhaps this sort of idea is in your mind:

'Well, I must say that I have been doing very well with smoking today. I haven't had a cigarette for two hours or more now. I'm making real progress. I didn't even feel like one with my cup of coffee! I went through that deprogramming thing very well. Well, I don't have to stop until D-Day, so I may as well have one now. It's about time . . .'

Patting yourself on the back? Flattery? Yes, a very clever rationalization, a very subtle trick to tempt you to smoke. It is so clever, that under the circumstances, you may very well go ahead and light up. However, it seems such a shame to think of rewarding yourself for being good with something that is actually slowly killing you!

You may also feel like this:

'I'm sick and tired of all this programming business. I feel confused about all the things you have to do. I'll just sit down and enjoy a smoke!' Would you like to know exactly how to deal with rationalizations? Read on.

Program 3

Program 3 is used to counteract rationalizations. If you deny yourself a cigarette, the immediate response of your body will be to tense up until you give it another nicotine fix, and your PCPs will start making up convincing reasons why you should light up.

Learn Program 3 by heart so that it will remind you to be aware of rationalizations and how to cope with them. This is how it goes:

PROGRAM 3

<u>E</u>ach day it is becoming easy   **E**
<u>A</u>nd my mind is becoming calm   **A**
<u>S</u>o there are no good reasons to smoke   **S**
<u>Y</u>esterday's craving is gone   **Y**

Spend time learning Program 3. It really is EASY to learn. The idea it contains will occur to you whenever you begin to make up excuses or false reasons to smoke. There are no good reasons to smoke, but your mind will continue to make up reasons why you should. Program 3 helps make you aware of what is actually happening, and helps remind you what to do about it – calm your restless mind.

You will probably be well aware already of your tension and rationalizations. They can be counteracted effectively by the same method, the meditation technique. So saying Program 3 reminds you of the need to meditate as soon as possible. In fact, you should aim to do so for 20 minutes at least once every day.

How Do I Calm My Restless Mind?

- Simply being aware of what is happening, being aware that your biocomputer will invent all sorts of reasons for you to smoke, and reasons why you shouldn't give up smoking will often turn the rationalization off. By being aware of the process at work, you can to some extent gain conscious control over what you are thinking about.

- Learn to distract yourself. If you consciously let your mind dwell on how much you really want a cigarette, or let yourself be drawn into a contest between the desire to have a cigarette and your desire to resist smoking (willpower), the desire to smoke will almost always win. Willpower is no match for the more powerful pro-cigarette programming. Rather than *fight* the desire to smoke, you can actually train yourself to distract your conscious attention away from smoking to something else. This is a particularly useful thing to do. If you can distract your attention with something else for only 60 seconds, the desire to smoke will pass. If you think that this technique of distracting your conscious attention away from smoking would be useful for you, practise it several times in your imagination. You will find that you are able to do it easily if you are willing to try it. It simply means consciously deciding to go and do something else, or occupy yourself with some activity for at least 60 seconds, until the desire to smoke has passed.

- Learn to meditate. This is the most powerful and effective way of stopping your mind from churning out rationalizations, and reminding you that you feel like smoking. It is so simple to learn and to use and has the great benefit that your body becomes very deeply relaxed, and you are able to unburden yourself of much of your tension. When you have learned to meditate, you should try and practise meditation for 20 minutes a day while you are giving up.

- If all else fails and you are unable to sit down for 20 minutes and meditate, and unable to distract your attention for 60 seconds, and you still feel like smoking, don't let yourself become more tense, upset or worried. Smoke a cigarette and say Program 1 to yourself while doing so! Smoke it deliberately and consciously, saying Program 1 in the same manner.

Breaking the Stress-Smoke Spiral

When smokers begin to cut down their consumption, they typically get caught up in a *stress-smoke spiral*. The less they smoke, the more tense or stressed they become. The more tense they become, the more they feel like smoking. This process can easily spiral a would-be non-smoker back into old smoking patterns again. In order to prevent this, and to allow the deprogramming/reprogramming process to completely eliminate smoking, you need to intervene and stop the stress-smoke spiral. To relieve the tension being built up in the body, the smoker must have a fix of nicotine which temporarily satisfies the urge to smoke. However, there are more satisfying and beneficial ways of relieving this tension and built-up stress. One of the most effective is meditation.

Meditation is an extremely simple and yet very valuable technique for producing profound relaxation and mental calm. Unlike tranquillizers, it has no side effects. Experiments have shown that the practice of meditation does indeed relieve stress, and meditators tend to be more calm and relaxed than non-meditators. It is also being used to treat hypertension and drug withdrawal programmes. By following the instructions below, you will be able to:

- dramatically reduce your desire to smoke
- reduce your tension level and break the *stress-smoke* spiral;
- deal more effectively with any stress from your work or family situation;
- lower your blood pressure if it is higher than it should be;
- really enjoy quitting smoking.

Learn the technique now, and practise it every day until you have completely stopped smoking. You will find that by using it you will be able to get through the period when the body readjusts to not having a constant inflow of nicotine (the withdrawal period), without being irritable and emotionally upset. It requires just 20 minutes a day to be highly effective, and is an enjoyable experience.

The technique which you will learn was developed by Dr Herbert Benson at the Beth Israel Hospital in Boston. It is quite similar to the 'Transcendental Meditation' publicized in the West by Maharishi Mahesh Yogi, who taught the Beatles how to meditate.

How To Meditate

In its simplest, most basic form, meditation has four essential requirements:

A Quiet Environment

Ideally you should choose a quiet calm room with as few distractions as possible. A quiet environment contributes to the effectiveness of the meditation by making it easier to eliminate distracting thoughts. When you do hear distracting noises, try not to let them upset you. Listen to them for a few moments, then gently go back to your meditation.

A Constant Mental Stimulus

To shift your mind from worrisome or negative thoughts, there should be a constant mental stimulus which you can repeat silently. Since the relaxation effect is caused by the mind becoming calm, the repetition of a word (or mantra) is a way to break a train of distracting thoughts or stop your mind wandering. Your eyes should remain closed. Attention to your normal breathing rhythm is also useful and enhances the repetition of the mantra, a sound or word you focus your mind on. A good example is the word 'relax'. Say it over and over: 'Relax . . . Relax . . . Relax.'

A Passive Attitude

When distracting thoughts occur (as they will), they are simply to be disregarded, and your attention redirected gently to the repetition of the mantra. This is really very simple to do. As soon as you become aware that you are thinking about something else, let your attention drift back to the word, without worrying about it. Don't force things – let yourself enjoy it. You should not worry about how well you are performing the technique, or worry whether or not you are doing it correctly, as then your attention will be on your worries, not on the mantra. If you start to worry about how well you are doing, treat it as just another thought, and gently redirect your attention to the mantra. Adopt a 'let it happen' attitude.

The passive attitude is perhaps the most important element for a relaxing meditation. Distracting thoughts may occur, but don't worry about them. They do not mean you are performing the technique incorrectly. When you realize that you are thinking about something else, just go back to repeating the word. Take it gently, and enjoy it.

A Comfortable Position

A comfortable position is important, so that there is no undue muscular tension at the outset. Your hands and arms are most relaxed when they are not crossed but lying comfortably in your lap. Allow your head to fall into a comfortable position. If you are lying down, you are more likely to fall asleep. You should be comfortable and relaxed in a sitting position.

Instructions

Before you begin to meditate, you should first read this section of the book, to help guide you into a relaxing meditation.

1 Sit quietly in a comfortable position.
2 Close your eyes and let your mind drift for a few minutes.
3 Deeply relax all your muscles, beginning at your feet and progressing up to your face. Keep them relaxed.
4 Breathe through your nose. Become aware of your breath-

ing. Breathe naturally and normally. Listen to the sound of your breathing.

5 As you become more relaxed and your breathing becomes more steady, as you breathe slowly out, say, 'I am becoming relaxed,' silently to yourself. Breathe in, breathe out: 'I am becoming relaxed.' As you progress more and more into a relaxed state, you need only repeat, 'Relax,' each time you breathe out. Breathe in, breathe out. 'Relax.'

6 Continue to meditate for 20 minutes. You may open your eyes to check the time on a clock or watch near you. There is no need to set the alarm.

7 When you finish, sit quietly for several minutes, at first with your eyes closed, and later with your eyes open. Try not to stand up for a few minutes.

8 Do not worry about whether or not you achieve a deep enough level of relaxation. Maintain a passive attitude and let relaxation occur at its own pace. When distracting thoughts occur, just let them pass by, and return easily to repeating, 'Relax.' The whole process should be perfectly effortless. There is no need to strain or force things. The more you allow it to just happen, the easier and more successfully you will be able to meditate. With practice, you will find that your body can relax very deeply without any effort.

9 Practise this technique as often as you like, but make sure you do it at least once each day for about 20 minutes.

10 If you use this technique regularly, for 20 minutes a day, you will be able to break the *stress-smoke spiral* by releasing tension in your body, and producing a calm state of mind.

The feelings associated with meditation are pleasurable. The more you enjoy it, the easier you will find it to relax deeply. Remember, just as each of us experiences anger, contentment and excitement, each of us has the capacity to experience the deep relaxation which meditation can provide.

James' Progress

By Thursday evening, James had smoked just six cigarettes so far that day, and felt very pleased. He was thinking about not going out with friends on Thursday night, as he did not want to spoil his success. However, he had been advised to carry out normal everyday activities while trying to stop, and he knew that going out for a drink on Thursday night was part of his weekly routine. So he went along to the pub with friends. His colleagues noticed the rubber band on James' cigarette packet and thought it was strange. James felt a sense of pride in describing this unheard-of method of quitting smoking. James used the card for the first cigarette that he smoked and recited the 'NURD' poem out loud in front of his colleagues. By his second cigarette, he was still using the rubber band. He did not note the following cigarettes on his card but he made a mental note and also told himself that the cigarettes were unpleasant and that he was losing the desire to smoke. He felt a genuine lack of desire to smoke that night. He smoked only eight cigarettes on Thursday.

Summary

- Use Program 1 every time you smoke.
- Use Program 2 every time you feel like smoking.
- Use Program 3 every time you invent reasons to smoke.
- You can calm your restless mind and reduce the tension in your body by using the meditation technique.
- You can calm your restless mind by becoming aware of what your mind is doing to you, and by distracting your conscious attention away from smoking.
- Don't get involved in a struggle between your desire to smoke and your desire to stop smoking. If you use willpower, you are likely to lose. Use the more subtle methods of meditation, relaxation and distraction.
- Complete your Daily Reduction Card and, at the end of the day, record the day's total on your Progress Chart.
- Enjoy the process of transforming yourself into a non-smoker!

Days 4, 5 and 6: Friday, Saturday and Sunday – Overcoming Unhelpful Thinking Patterns

By this point, you should be well on the way to becoming a happy and successful non-smoker. If you have been following all of the procedures described in Chapters three to five, your enjoyment of smoking will be considerably reduced and you will be smoking much less often than previously. However, it is still important that you continue to smoke whenever you feel like having a cigarette and that you say Program 1 (NURD) to yourself while you smoke it. This eliminates the pleasure PCPs in your brain that tell you that smoking is enjoyable. It will remind your body of the true effects of smoking, which you experienced the first time you ever smoked.

It is essential that you also continue to Stop, Think, and Deprogram using Program 2 (WEST-D). This will eliminate the automatic way in which your smoking triggers make you light up every time they occur. You do not really want to be like a robot that automatically responds every time a smoking-related stimulus appears in your environment. Give yourself strong verbal commands that you will smoke only when you choose to do so. You do not simply have to smoke just because one of your triggers dictates that you must immediately have a smoke.

While Programs 1 and 2 will continue to work for you as you reduce your consumption, you should also allow time for Program 3 (EASY). Both imagery rehearsal and meditation take a little time, but they will both have a very calming effect on your mind. By now, you should have discovered the extra confidence that imagery rehearsal can bring you in reprogramming triggers. You should also have experienced the restful and relaxing effects that a few minutes' meditation can bring. The days that immediately precede D-Day are very crucial ones. These are the final days remaining to deprogram and reprogram your automatic triggers. The weekend days often present triggers that are different from those that you experience during the weekdays. Please be on the lookout, then, for some new triggers. You also need to be on the lookout for the subtle and seductive process of *rationalization*. Rationalization is represented by a process which I call the Argument Game. This is a fight that breaks out between the Smoker in you and the Non-smoker that is trying to break free.

Smoker Versus Non-smoker

It is at this stage that imagery rehearsal and meditation can be most beneficial. This is because there will be some very strong rationalizations operating as the battle heats up between your two *alter egos*, 'Smoker' and 'Non-smoker', who by now are definitely not seeing eye to eye. As predicted, the less you smoke, the more Smoker will struggle to generate good reasons why you should continue to smoke. As the deprogramming and reprogramming produces some positive results and your consumption of tobacco goes down, the more desperate Smoker will become. He or she is hell-bent on keeping you smoking and will try all kinds of psychological tricks to mask the true facts of the situation. Be prepared. Do not be conned as he or she tries to make smoking as attractive as possible to your conscious mind.

Non-smoker knows that smoking is a filthy, stinking, lethal habit. Smoker, on the other hand, tells you that smoking is a relaxing, satisfying, and safe pastime. This internal 'Argument Game' continues almost constantly when you try to stop smoking by the use of willpower. In this CBT programme, it has been one of the main aims to keep the use of willpower to minimum levels. However, the Argument Game continues, and it is essential that Non-smoker learns how to win.

According to Smoker, statistics are all a pack of lies – there is no evidence that smoking kills, it is purely statistical, nobody knows the cause of cancer, and that's why there isn't any cure. Smoker will tempt you with all kinds of safe-sounding propositions such as: 'Go on, have one. You've only had three today and it's nearly bedtime. Have one now; it's only fair. You've done so well, you deserve a small reward.' Small reward, indeed! That's precisely the kind of nonsense that's kept smokers hooked for generations.

Another deceptive little ruse is the 'It won't happen to me' syndrome. This is so well known to psychologists that it has been given a special name, 'unrealistic optimism'. Everybody thinks that bad things won't happen to *them*, only to others. Of course, when something bad does happen, there is always the plaintive question: 'Why me?' The 'Not Me/Why Me?' illusion is practically universal in situations where people indulge in risky activities. Because they are doing it by choice, they feel a false sense of personal control over what the outcome will be. The fact is that lung cancer doesn't care why the victims' lungs are so crammed full of nasty toxic substances, it simply spreads and spreads until they require treatment or die.

In this chapter you will be guided to learn Program 4. This technique enables you to combat the rationalizations which your old pro-cigarette programming churns out and you can avoid getting involved in a power struggle between the two parts of your self. You will learn how to anticipate some of the more common rationalizations. These are pseudo-reasons for having a cigarette, generated by your biocomputer or which you may hear other smokers saying when they hear that you're trying to give up. This technique plays the Argument Game and gives every extra advantage to Non-smoker that it possibly can.

Program 4

Learn the following Program which will triumph over the bio-computer's last stand, the Argument Game.

PROGRAM 4	
<u>N</u>o matter what you say	**N**
There's <u>o</u>nly <u>o</u>ne way	**O**
To play The Argument <u>G</u>ame	**G**
There are <u>no</u> good reasons to smoke	**O**

Learn Program 4 by heart (NO GO). It reflects the only sane attitude you can adopt as your biocomputer starts to send you its Phoney Pro-Cigarette Arguments (PPCAs) – you just tell it NO GO!

Spend some time now reading through the ten PPCAs below, and the ten counter-arguments that go with them. Become familiar with the counter-arguments so that you will be able to use them when needed. You should then be able to completely deflate these common rationalizations whenever they occur. Have the counter-arguments ready so that you can say them either in response to your own biocomputer or to other smokers. Knowing what to say can make all the difference. Non-smoker will be strengthened and Smoker weakened by pure good sense, logic and scientific evidence! The rational use of information is rarely sufficient by itself as a method for stopping smoking. However, when you use cold logic in combination with your emotions and motivation, you have a total package which Smoker will find impossible to defeat.

Remember, there are absolutely no good reasons to smoke. Absolutely none! However, as Non-smoker takes over control, Smoker will become even more subtle and devious. It may try to tempt you to stop following the QUIT FOR LIFE Programme, it may tell you that things are completely hopeless, or that it is really too late to stop now because the damage has already been done or that you wouldn't get cancer anyway.

Ten Phoney Pro-cigarette Arguments and Their Counter-arguments

Rationalizations fall into four main categories:

1 Health
2 Social Pressure
3 Economic
4 Personal Discomfort

Study the Phoney Pro-Cigarette Arguments very carefully. These, or similar ones, may be lurking in your mind right now. If you become aware of them, use counter-arguments to eliminate them. This process is not intended to be a way of strengthening your willpower. Nor does it eliminate the need to continue what you have already started to do. Whenever you feel like a smoke, it is important to smoke, but use Programs 1 and 2 while doing so. The Argument Game is a way of noticing what is going on and tackling the phoniness of Smoker's case head on.

Health

Typically these arguments emerge in the company of other smokers. They feel threatened when they see that you are giving up the habit and trot out arguments of the following kind:

Phoney Pro-cigarette Argument 1
All the evidence linking smoking with lung cancer is only statistical and has no relevance to me.

Counter-Argument 1
A series of reports published by the Royal College of Physicians in England has been categorical in stating that the simplest explanation of the evidence showing a relationship between smoking and lung cancer is *causal*. It is the view of all the major

medical authorities that smoking cigarettes causes lung cancer. Smoking is known to be the largest single preventable cause of mortality and it accounts for one-third of all deaths in middle age (40 to 64 years). In addition to causing 90 per cent of all lung cancers, nearly all of which are fatal, smoking also produces cancer of the mouth, larynx, pharynx, oesophagus, pancreas, bladder, and other organs. In fact, smoking causes more premature deaths than AIDS, cocaine, heroin, alcohol, fire, car accidents, homicide, and suicide put together! The more you smoke, and the longer the time you spend as a smoker, the greater the risk of developing cancer or the many other diseases which are caused by smoking, such as chronic bronchitis, emphysema, and coronary heart disease. The sooner a person stops smoking, the lower the chances of contracting one of these terrible diseases.

Phoney Pro-Cigarette Argument 2

OK, I accept the evidence that smoking is harmful to my health but it really is too late now. The damage has probably already been done. There's little point in carrying on with this programme as it only adds to my worries. I thought it was a good idea to try and give up when I first started, but it's too much effort, especially when it's probably too late to do anything anyway.

Counter-Argument 2

Reports from The Royal College of Physicians in the UK and 28 Surgeon General's Reports on Smoking and Health, 1964–2004, in the US, have shown a reduced risk of cancer among those who stop smoking. The risk of lung cancer could be cut in half within two or three years after cigarette smoking is stopped. The 2004 Surgeon General's report concluded that quitting smoking has immediate and long-term benefits, reducing risks for diseases caused by smoking and improving health in general. 'Within minutes and hours after smokers inhale that last cigarette, their bodies begin a series of changes that continue for years,' the Surgeon General Dr Richard H.

Carmona stated. 'Among these health improvements are a drop in heart rate, improved circulation, and reduced risk of heart attack, lung cancer and stroke. By quitting smoking today a smoker can assure a healthier tomorrow.'

Dr Carmona has stated that 'It is never too late to stop smoking. Quitting smoking at age 65 or older reduces a person's risk of dying of a smoking-related disease by nearly 50 per cent.' Within a few days of smoking you will actually feel a lot better. You will feel fitter, breathe more easily, lose the frog in your throat, and regain your senses of smell and taste that are partly shut off by smoking. You will also smell a lot cleaner and fresher without the stink of stale tobacco smoke on your clothes, hair, and skin. The sooner you give up, the sooner your physical health will return to normal levels.

Recent research has shown that giving up smoking has a positive effect on reducing the risk of coronary heart disease (CHD), regardless of age. The relative risks of CHD were compared in never-smokers, former-smokers and current smokers in men of two age groups, 51 to 59 and 65 to 74. In both age groups there was a consistent decrease in CHD incidence as smoking experience decreased, and former-smokers in both age groups showed lower incidence of CHD than smokers. Thus, quitting smoking, even at an advanced age, results in a reduction of risk. It is never too late to quit smoking.

Phoney Pro-Cigarette Argument 3

OK, I accept that I'll be healthier physically, but I depend on cigarettes to perk me up, to help me relax and to concentrate. I won't be able to perform as well when under pressure if I can't have a cigarette.

Counter-Argument 3

It is true that smoking is perceived as a stimulating and relaxing thing to do. However good you may feel when you have a cigarette, you know that this is one of the main effects of the dependency that you have built up. By deprogramming your desire to smoke and by learning new ways of relaxing, you will be able to cope with pressure and stress much better without the need to have a smoke. You will also be able to concentrate on what you are doing without the need for a cigarette.

A cigarette only seems necessary at present because your central nervous system has become used to having regular supplies of nicotine. You are a cigarette junkie who needs a regular hit of nicotine. As a smoker you perceive that smoking helps alleviate your negative mood states, but the evidence from the Royal College of Physicians suggests that 'the only negative mood state so alleviated is that resulting directly from the nicotine dependence itself. Thus, the nicotine in tobacco relieves nicotine withdrawal symptoms, but does not have mood enhancing properties in non-addicted individuals. If anything, the experience of being addicted to tobacco appears to add to, rather than relieve, stress in the everyday lives of smokers.' (In other words, you are rationalizing and justifying your smoking, using a false argument. Smoking makes you want to smoke more. It is only calming because you are addicted.)

Social Pressure

Phoney Pro-Cigarette Argument 4

Other smokers, or even your own biocomputer, may churn out the following: But I've heard about people who've been smokers and lived to 90, and then there are others who've never smoked and die in their 40s. You die when you die and that's all there is to it. At least you may as well be happy while you're alive.

Counter-Argument No. 4

People who use these sorts of arguments ought to study Counter-Arguments 1 to 3. Try to avoid arguments with other smokers. Simply tell them, 'No, thanks. But you go ahead if you want to.' Social pressure takes many different forms. It was probably social pressure that helped to get you smoking in the first place. Don't let these pressures affect you again, now that you are aware of the facts about smoking. If others want to smoke, that is really their affair, and you certainly do not need to keep them company. Tell yourself (and your biocomputer) that you will make a point of refusing when others put pressure on you to smoke. Compared to ten or fifteen years ago, the tables have turned and there is a lot of pressure on smokers to stop smoking. As an almost non-smoker, you can therefore easily take the upper hand. Be assertive and say, 'No, thank you,' every time you're offered a smoke by another person. It won't be long before all your smoking friends will want to follow your example and give up too. Be proud, firm, and confident, and always say no.

Phoney Pro-Cigarette Argument 5
In spite of Counter-Argument 4 above, your biocomputer, or another smoker, may eventually push you to the limit and say: 'Go on, have one. One cigarette can't do you any harm.' Initially, you may even feel like giving in by thinking or even saying, 'That's right. Just one can't make much difference. I'll just have this one.'

Counter-Argument 5

How dangerous the Argument Game is becoming! Especially so if you start agreeing with devious Smoker and all its phoney arguments. Don't be a fool! This is the oldest trick in the book. When you stop to think about it, every smoking habit consists of one long series of 'Just one' cigarettes. When you find the Argument Game turning into the Just One Game, you know you've still got some serious deprogramming to do. If you do have 'just one', remember always to say Program 1. And, every time you feel like one, use the WEST-D procedure at the same time.

Another version of the Just One Game has already been mentioned. This is when your biocomputer congratulates you for being so clever in cutting down and then suggests that you deserve a cigarette as a reward! This is surprisingly common, so be on your guard at all times. The old Smoker programs would love to catch you out because Smoker realizes that 'just one' cigarette wouldn't be just one at all, but a whole new series of cigarettes, and then the full-blown habit would quickly become re-established. You wouldn't fall for this one now – or would you?

Phoney Pro-Cigarette Argument 6
Somebody you are close to may be a smoker and perhaps you're trying to stop, but they are not. The person (X) says to you: 'Come on, have a cigarette.' Or you watch them smoking and your biocomputer says, 'Go on, have one. If you don't, X will start sulking. No point in creating a fuss. You'll get along together if you don't rock the boat by refusing to smoke.'

Counter-Argument 6
However appealing this tugging at your heart-strings may be, it is of course a false reason for smoking. Your eventual success at giving up will provide an excellent incentive for your partner to follow suit. Ideally, both of you will be giving up at the same time. Never smoke because somebody else does. There are no good reasons to smoke.

Economic

These arguments are perhaps the weakest and flimsiest of them all. However, your biocomputer, under the influence of your pro-cigarette programming, will try any argument at all to try to get you smoking again.

Phoney Pro-Cigarette Argument 7
Your biocomputer says: 'You gave up smoking because you thought you'd notice it in your pocket. But you haven't really saved much cash. What have you got to show for it so far in hard cash? For what you save, it's hardly worth the effort to give up.'

Counter-Argument 7

Calculate your own personal life expenditure on cigarettes. Some people have used what they would formerly have spent on cigarettes to buy something they have wanted for a long time. One woman used the £25.00 she used to spend per week on cigarettes to pay off a washing machine and dryer (and she still had £10.00 extra money). Think how much you will save.

Rosemary used to smoke a packet of cigarettes a day before she stopped. In 2004, just before she stopped, she was spending £4.70 per day, or £32.90 per week, on cigarettes. Multiplying this by 52 gives a total of over £1,700 per year. Since Rosemary was paying tax at 25 pence in the pound, smoking was costing her £2,280 per year of gross income.

Make your own calculation. See how much smoking was costing you:

Cost per day: _____
Cost per week: _____
Cost per year: _____

Now decide what you'd like to do with your extra money. Think of something which you could purchase. How about some new clothes, a special trip, new DVD player, camcorder, dishwasher, or a surprise present for someone special? Work out now what you will do with the money you save by continuing life as a non-smoker.

Personal Discomfort

For many people, the discomfort caused by restlessness, depression or ill-tempered moods and nervous habits seem to be a big problem. This collection of discomforts is what psychologists and doctors call *withdrawal symptoms*. Some people find that their consumption of snacks, such as nuts, ice cream and soft drinks increases when they cut down on cigarettes. Your bio-computer can easily manipulate you into this vulnerable situation. Beware of threats about might happen to you when you stop.

Phoney Pro-Cigarette Argument No. 8

Your biocomputer may suggest: 'Think how terrible you will feel if you stop smoking.'

Counter-Argument No. 8

For the first few days, or at most weeks, the smoker who does not relax may well feel moody and ill at ease. But, however you feel at this stage, it is infinitely more bearable than cancer, bronchitis, or emphysema, where your lungs are actually eroded away. However awful, irritable, or ill-tempered you may feel, the long-term gains are well worth the effort. Your bio-computer may try and convince you that you are losing control, and that to start smoking again is your only solution, your only way of returning to normal. These are powerful and persuasive arguments, but they are wrong. Smoking is certainly not normal, and you are gaining control, not losing it, when you quit smoking.

If you allow yourself to relax deeply, by meditating, and use mental rehearsal to reprogram the rest of your triggers, you can avoid the discomfort of built-up tension during the withdrawal stage.

Phoney Pro-Cigarette Argument No. 9

This argument is very similar to number 8, so watch out for it! Your biocomputer (or an interested bystander) says: 'If you stop smoking you will gain unwanted weight. If you carry on smoking, you will stay slim.'

Counter-Argument No. 9

Your biocomputer is trying to flatter you by appealing to your vanity. But, rest assured, if you put on a few extra pounds now, it will be worthwhile. First, stopping smoking will give you a happier, healthier life in the long run. Second, in a few weeks you will be able to normalize your weight without using smoking as a form of weight control. Your long-term health is surely more important than a little extra weight in the short term. At the moment, smoking is the problem you should focus on. You can tackle the weight problem, if it develops, later; see Chapter eight for more details.

Phoney Pro-Cigarette Argument 10
Your biocomputer says: 'You have already cut down on your consumption. That's good enough. There's no need to go any further. Your lower daily consumption is a fine achievement. Well done. Have a cigarette. Just one cigarette won't do you any harm'.

Counter-Argument 10
The Just One Game is a crafty trick played by your biocomputer under the last remnants of its control. Your PCPs have all but disappeared and they are desperately trying to regain their lost control. Your goal is to give up smoking completely. You know all the reasons. If you pretend you are satisfied with yourself by continuing to smoke at your current daily level, then think again. Your smoking will easily creep up to the original level; your biocomputer and pro-cigarette programming will have beaten you; and, once more, you will be a smoker.

The path is clear and obvious: never, ever succumb to an argument which tells you to give in. You will not be content until you have given up smoking completely and forever.

This list of Pro-Cigarette Arguments and Counter-Arguments could be extended. By now you should be able to recognize the Argument Game, and be well prepared to deal with any Pro-Cigarette Argument which comes along. Remember, there are absolutely no good reasons to smoke.

Systematic Sensitization Using the Eight Steps

You are now very close to D-Day, the day when you will not smoke. If you have been following this therapy programme carefully, you will have most of the automatic responses you have experienced as a smoker under your control. On D-Day, you will find it easy to maintain your self-control and do what you consciously desire to do – not to smoke.

However, you are very well aware of the power of the programs in your mind, which continue to put pressure on you to smoke. There will be times when you are tempted to have a cigarette. There will be situations which trigger the desire to smoke, which you have been unable to deprogram because they have not come up yet. There may be times on D-Day or afterwards when your biocomputer (under the influence of a PCP) will suggest that you 'Just have one puff" or 'Just have one last one', or 'Just have a few puffs to see if you really do or don't like smoking any more'. It could play the Just One Game for some considerable time.

The next section provides a further technique to help you finally destroy your dying PCPs. By using it, you should be able to calmly resist having that 'Just One', even if you are really tempted. Your success is obviously going to be linked to being able to stay calm and in control of yourself without having to force yourself by using your willpower. By using willpower, you open up the conflict between two competing desires: the desire to smoke and the desire to stop smoking. It is usually far easier to smoke than to fight. You must constantly be on your guard and employ more powerful methods of defence than argument alone. The technique that follows is a way of sensitizing you to the true effects of smoking, and will remind your body of the true effects of smoking.

To use the sensitization technique to full advantage, you should read the next section right through. Use your creative imagination to link each step with the visual image suggested. Treat this technique seriously, and follow the instructions exactly. You may find the imagery rather disturbing. However, the descriptions accurately reflect the realities of smoking. By avoiding these situations, you are closing your eyes to what actually happens when people smoke. Have a packet of cigarettes handy before you read on. Be encouraged by the fact that this packet could be your last!

The Eight Steps

Please acquaint yourself fully with the Eight Steps. Although it is possible that you are not consciously aware of them, you go through them every time you smoke. Take a few minutes now to learn the Eight Steps.

STEP 1: Pick up the packet , open it and look at the cigarettes inside. Be aware of how the cigarettes look. Do it now.

STEP 2: Take a cigarette out of the packet, but don't put it in your mouth yet. Become aware of what it feels like to hold the cigarette between your fingers. Roll it around a little to really get the feel of it.

STEP 3: Put the cigarette in your mouth. You should become aware of the sensation between your lips. Do it now. Really try to experience the shape and the feel of the cigarette in your lips.

STEP 4: Now light a match or lighter. Bring the flame up almost to the end of the cigarette, but don't light it. You will actually feel the heat of the flame on your face and fingers. Become aware of the heat from the flame on the surface of your skin.

STEP 5: Now light the cigarette and inhale a puff of smoke. Be aware of the smoke you inhale.

STEP 6: Now exhale the smoke from the first puff. Feel it and see it coming out of your mouth.

STEP 7: Smoke the cigarette through. Of course, don't forget to use Program 1 as you smoke it.

STEP 8: Stub out the cigarette in the ashtray. This time, stub it out rather more forcefully than normal. You are aware of the pressure on your thumb or fingers as you stub it out.

Linking The Eight Steps To Visual Images

In this section we will use the eight steps and link a visual image to each of them. As you read this section through, really try to visualize each situation. The association will be so powerful that, each time you go to have a cigarette, you will automatically think of the image you have linked with it. The association will be so strong, that you will have an automatic warning device to help you overcome the temptation to have a cigarette. Remember that the desire to smoke is only a trick of the mind conjured up by your biocomputer to force you to administer yourself a fix of nicotine. By using this sensitization technique, you will have a whole series of warnings, which will remind you that you are being tricked into smoking. You will reprogram your biocomputer with new anti-smoking programs to replace the diminishing traces of your old pro-smoking programs.

Be prepared now to *smoke a cigarette in your mind*. You are going to create a fantasy experience by imagining that you are lighting a cigarette while you are reading. As you read, try to imagine that you are going through the procedure of lighting and smoking a cigarette. Do this as vividly and realistically as you possibly can.

STEP 1: Your packet of cigarettes is lying beside you. You decide to have a cigarette. You pick up the packet and open the lid. As the lid opens, and you look into the packet, you see not cigarettes, but the dead bodies of people who have died from lung cancer. Imagine that each cigarette is one dead body wrapped in a white sheet. The cigarette packet you are holding is a coffin full of cancer victims who died because they were cigarette smokers.

STEP 2: Now imagine that you take a cigarette out of the packet. You are aware of its shape. It turns into a bottle of lethal poison, which you are going to administer to yourself. It is a paper container filled with dozens of cancer-producing chemicals. You are now going to take this brew of lethal poisons into your system – a form of slow-motion suicide.

STEP 3: Imagine that you now put the cigarette into your mouth. You are aware of it between your lips. You feel the roundness of the filter; you are very aware of the unpleasantness this causes in you because it almost seems as if there is a cancerous growth on your lip. You can feel it on your lip growing and spreading. It is a cancer caused by cigarette smoking, a cancer which occurs substantially more often in smokers than in non-smokers. You can feel it between your lips.

STEP 4: Now imagine that you light a match or your cigarette lighter. You look at the flame, at the fire and, as you bring it closer to your face, you become very aware of the heat on the surface of your skin. You can feel the heat, the fire on your face. You think to yourself, this is the fire I am going to take into my lungs. This is the burning fire which will destroy me.

STEP 5: Imagine that you light the cigarette. Imagine that you are very tiny and that you are standing inside your own mouth. You can see your teeth, tongue and, as you look around, you become aware of your lips. Between your lips you can see the round end of the cigarette sticking through into your mouth. You hear a rumbling sound as your chest, far below, begins to expand and you begin to breathe. As your chest expands, you suddenly see the thick grey-white smoke pour out of the end of the cigarette. It is thick and dense. It pours into your mouth, and as you watch, you can see the tiny droplets of thick brown, oozing tar being deposited onto your teeth; you can see the dense white smoke pour down the opening at the back of your mouth into the throat. It pours, rushes down, down through your larynx, down the tubes which lead into your lungs. You can see the tiny hairs covered with mucus on the inside of the tubes freeze. Their function as the dirt removal system of the lungs is paralyzed. You can see the dense smoke enter the tiny air sacs of your lungs. You can see the droplets of tar being deposited on the delicate tissues of your lungs. You are very aware that the whole atmosphere inside your breathing system is filled with poisonous gases. Hydrogen cyanide – one of the deadliest gases known, used as a poison gas during World War I. Nitrogen dioxide – the amount of this gas in one cigarette can produce an acid strong enough to burn holes in a nylon stocking; this is the gas which may cause emphysema, where the tiny air sacs burst and collapse in the body's struggle to obtain oxygen and get rid of carbon monoxide. Carbon monoxide – a gas which is quickly absorbed into the bloodstream, and is swiftly transported to the brain, where it begins to cause substantial impairment of its function. It starts to impair your vision, judgement and attentiveness to sounds. The smoke, the gases: you are suffocating, you are suffocating!

STEP 6: You are now aware of movements in your diaphragm, which now begins to push upwards, to push the smoke out of the lungs. You feel the movement of the diaphragm; it is almost the same sensation you feel when you are sick, and begin to vomit. As the diaphragm pushes upwards, the smoke begins to spew out of your mouth; it is as if your body can no longer tolerate the poisonous fumes. It is forcing them out, almost vomiting them out.

STEP 7: You continue to draw on the cigarette, and the smoke continues to pour down your lungs. You are very aware of the effects of the smoke on your body. You are reciting Program 1 to yourself. You can feel the heat of the smoke on your tongue, feel the harshness on your throat; you can feel your heart pumping harder than normal because, from the first puff you took, the drug nicotine began to speed it up and put a strain on it. You can feel the strain on your heart. You continue to smoke the cigarette down to the hot, bitter end.

STEP 8:   You feel ill; you feel the heaviness, the thickness, the aching in your head. You can tolerate it no more – you cannot, you *will* not tolerate it any more. You stub it out hard, killing it before it kills you.

If you feel at all tense or upset for any reason after reading this section, make use of the strong feelings you have to continue deprogramming yourself of the desire to smoke. Say to yourself, 'I have had it with smoking! I just don't want to smoke any more. I refuse to be pushed into something that I don't really want to do.' Spend a few minutes now, giving your biocomputer some very strong *verbal commands* about how you want to see yourself. Do this now! It is worth the effort to spend a few moments talking to yourself in a strong and definite way. When you have finished giving yourself some strong verbal commands about how you want to be completely free from cigarette smoking, take some time to relax. It will be very beneficial to you to spend 20 minutes meditating, just letting the tension flow out of your body. Sit back and let yourself completely relax.

Planning Your D-Day

This is the day that you will stop smoking. Choosing the right day for D-Day is crucial. D-Day is decision day but, just as importantly, so is the day immediately before D-Day. Coincidentally, I write this chapter 60 years to the day after the original D-Day (which was a Tuesday). I am able to say with some conviction that the planning of D-Day is absolutely crucial to its success. Just as more than 150,000 courageous people fought on the beaches of Normandy to free the world from the scourge of Hitler's Nazism, you and thousands of others can be free from the smoking scourge by fighting a carefully planned D-Day of your own.

Like our heroic forebears led by Churchill and Eisenhower, you need to decide which day is to be your D-Day, as much in advance as possible. At the very latest this will be during the

24-hour period immediately before. If you decide on one day but the weather is stormy (as it was way back on 5 June 1944), you can decide to delay it to another day when you will be confident enough to weather the stormy seas that will release you from the smoking habit.

For example, if you originally planned to make D-Day a Monday, then you may decide to make Tuesday your D-Day. What you should not do is decide to make Tuesday your D-Day on Tuesday. This is because you won't be sufficiently prepared, and part of Tuesday will already have gone. D-Day is a complete 24-hour period, starting at midnight and planned at least 24 hours in advance.

Here are a few guidelines, based on the experience of several thousand people who have already succeeded.

- Look at your Progress Chart. This will tell you exactly how well you are doing. Provisionally choose a day when you can be reasonably sure that your consumption will only be 1 to 3 cigarettes on D-Day Minus One. The trend could be something like this:
  - Tuesday: 24 cigarettes
  - Wednesday: 13 cigarettes
  - Thursday: 7 cigarettes
  - Friday: 4 cigarettes (set D-Day provisionally for Sunday)
  - Saturday: 2 cigarettes (confirm that D-Day will be Sunday
  - Sunday = D-Day: 0 cigarettes.
- When you arrive at D-Day Minus One, your cigarette consumption will hopefully be right on target and you will smoke only 1 to 3 cigarettes that day. In that case, your D-Day should be confirmed as definitely the next day. Make a deliberate, conscious decision, taking all factors into account. You should make the decision before midnight.
- Your consumption immediately prior to D-Day should be the main factor, but it is not the only one. Please also take into account what you will be doing that day. Choose a day

when you know things will be reasonably normal and quiet. Choose a day when you feel confident that you will succeed. Not everybody progresses as smoothly as shown in the example. Some people reduce their consumption and then have a bad day or two, when their smoking increases to higher levels again. In this case, follow the original procedures again, but apply more concentration to the de- and reprogramming while using Programs 1 to 4. Nobody who applies Programs 1 to 4 consistently should fail to reduce their cigarette consumption to zero. When your consumption has fallen to 1 to 2 cigarettes, which it should do within 5 to 10 days, then you know that your D-Day has arrived.

James' Progress

On Friday James smoked only six cigarettes. He went through the NOGO procedure and discovered a lot of rationalizing going on. More triggers also appeared that had not appeared earlier in the week. He realized that the weekend might bring some surprising new triggers and so he doubled his efforts to become aware of his inner thoughts and feelings as these seemed more relevant now than earlier in the week.

James learned the Eight Steps and when he smoked he not only used Program 1 (NURD) but he imagined the unpleasant images of each of the Eight Steps of smoking. James set aside a 20-minute quiet period on Saturday and Sunday for meditation. James gained a lot from this as he felt more calm and relaxed.

On Saturday James smoked five cigarettes and on Sunday James smoked only two cigarettes. He decided to make Tuesday his D-Day. On making the decision James felt he was making a 'new start' to his life. He resolved never to smoke again after midnight on Monday.

Summary

- Every time you smoke, think of the Eight Steps and the eight images that go with them.

- Continue using Programs 1 to 3 whenever or wherever the need arises.
- Meditate every day and practise mental rehearsal every night before you go to sleep.
- Become aware of all your biocomputer's rationalizations and play and win the Argument Game (Program 4: NO GO).
- Plan your D-Day carefully. Set yourself a target date. Confirm it the day before, when your consumption should be no more than 1–2 cigarettes. A well executed D-Day will free you from the scourge of smoking forever. Be a hero on your D-Day!
- Complete your Daily Reduction Card, and, at the end of the day, record the day's total on your Progress Chart.

7

Surviving D-Day and Starting Your New Life as a Non-smoker

Using the techniques in the last few chapters, you are now well equipped with some powerful methods for stopping smoking. Using these methods should be enough for most smokers to beat the smoking habit forever. This chapter gives you further techniques to finalize the process of quitting over the weekend and to help you to survive your D-Day.

This chapter should be consulted whenever you feel like a cigarette from D-Day onwards. If you do get the desire to smoke, there will always be something you can do about it. This chapter provides you with a variety of techniques to prevent any further smoking, however sorely you may be tempted. In Part Three, you will find details of other, longer-term ways of coping.

Here is a list of things that you can do on D-Day to get rid of any remaining desire to smoke:

Progressive Relaxation of Your Whole Body

Sit in a comfortable chair, with both feet resting on the floor and your hands in your lap. Close your eyes and, starting at your feet, gradually move up through your body, relaxing all of your muscles. Do this for your feet, calves, thighs, buttocks, back, shoulders, stomach, chest, shoulders, arms, hands, fingers, neck, face, mouth, eyes, cheeks, and forehead. Think of each area and say to yourself, 'My arms are relaxing, my arms are relaxing,' or, 'My face is relaxing, my face is relaxing.' Sit for a few minutes, doing this, and you will find that the physical relaxation of your body flows through into your mind.

This technique of deep relaxation can be most beneficial. You will be able to use it to change your self-concept to that of a non-smoker and experience a calm and confident feeling that you have crossed the boundary from being a smoker to becoming a non-smoker. Your mind will be freed from distractions and be more ready to accept new ideas and information. You will discover that your confidence is growing so that you will be able to strengthen your new non-smoking behaviour.

Meditation Exercise

Do this at least once on your D-Day, preferably early in the day before you encounter too many people, situations, or events. This exercise will relax you deeply and leave you feeling more calm and confident. It will strengthen your resolve and determination not to smoke. It will further weaken your automatic responses to triggers when you encounter them during the day. Your mind will become calm and you will be able to cope better with any remaining anxiety, stress, and strain that may bother you on D-Day. You should do this later in the day as well, if possible: in the afternoon, perhaps.

Fantasy Techniques

There are many of these, and you should be able to construct some of your own using the ideas listed below. The basic principle is to imagine pleasant scenes and situations which you know would make you feel perfectly calm and relaxed. For example, sit in your most comfortable chair, close your eyes, and imagine that you are lying on a beautiful beach in some exotic place in the warmth of the afternoon sun. Create a fantasy which allows you to feel at ease and comfortable. Let the pleasant scene unfold and, as it does so, you will feel very calm and relaxed.

Imagery Rehearsal

Follow the procedures described in Chapter five. While relaxed, imagine yourself in one of the trigger situations that you most fear. See it, hear it and feel it with all the powers of your imagination. Then imagine coping with this situation perfectly well without a cigarette. Remember, the more clearly and vividly you can imagine yourself coping with the problem situation, the more easily you will be able to manage it in real life. Repeat with other triggers, until you feel that you are capable of treating each of your triggers with complete detachment.

Body Imagery

Sit down and close your eyes. Imagine you can actually see your blood flow. Imagine your skin has suddenly turned transparent and you can see the flow of blood in your body, warm and cosy, bathing the muscles with a soothing relaxing effect. Imagine the warmth creeping up from your feet. Feel how comfortably warm your body is getting. Warmth in your legs, your abdomen, your chest. Warmth in your face. Feel the flow of warmth moving down your back. Continue for as long as you wish, then open your eyes.

Rag Doll Imagery

Sit down for a few minutes and close your eyes. Imagine you are a rag doll – a floppy soft rag doll that just collapses when dropped. A rag doll that straggles all over the place when you throw it down. Imagine that's what you are now. Throw your arms and legs out and let them just flop. Limp and floppy. See your rag doll muscles. They're made of wool. Limp, floppy wool! It is a ridiculous thought, but stay with it for a few minutes. Visualize your muscles dropping down there like a handful of wool. Repeat these images until you feel perfectly relaxed. Open your eyes.

Elevator Imagery

Sit down and close your eyes. Imagine that you are on the twentieth floor of a tall building. Imagine yourself going to the elevator. See yourself pressing the call button. See the elevator doors opening. Get into the elevator; see the doors closing. Now try and remember the feeling or sensation you get when an elevator begins to move down. Imagine yourself moving slowly and smoothly downwards. See the numbers light up as you go down. Say to yourself, 'As I go down, I feel more relaxed.' Say it every time you pass a floor. When you reach the ground floor, get out of the elevator, and relax for a short while. Then get back into the elevator and swiftly return to the twentieth floor and open your eyes.

Create A Space

This technique can be used at any time, whether you are with people or by yourself. It is extremely useful to be able to create a space in situations where you can't leave to sit down and relax. This is how to create a space:

(a) Select a time and place when you were particularly happy and relaxed. It may be a pleasant childhood memory, something that happened on your last trip, or the last time you were at the beach or in the country. The most important point is that you were feeling happy and relaxed, having a good time and enjoying yourself.

(b) If you can't think of a real experience, then make one up. Make it a beautiful experience. Perhaps it is in the mountains. Perhaps it's a very special dream.

(c) You must experience your situation. Try to remember or make up as many details as possible. Try to answer the following questions in your mind:
   • Where are you?
   • What time of day is it?

- What are you doing?
- Who is with you?
- What are you wearing?
- What are you touching?
- What colours are there?
- What can you see to the right and to the left?
- If you turn around, what can you see?
- Are you aware of any smells? (Flowers? The sea?)
- What is the weather like?
- Are you aware of any sounds? (Waves, birds, people, the wind?)
- Imagine how you are feeling.
- What were you doing half an hour ago?
- What are you likely to be doing in half an hour's time?

(d) Now that you have built up your fantasy in detail, you can begin to use it. Try now, in your imagination, to put yourself in that situation. Close your eyes for a minute and really visualize yourself there. Have a good look around your imaginary world, your very own space that you have created.

(e) Now come back to the situation in reality. Be aware of the things around you, and where you are.

(f) Practise shifting backwards and forwards into fantasy and back into reality.

(g) Now be very aware of the situation you are in. The real world. With your eyes open, imagine you are bringing your fantasy space into the real world. Imagine you are putting it on, like a suit of clothes. Perhaps you can imagine yourself enclosed in a bubble which contains that peaceful situation.

(h) Practise putting it on, and taking it off. All you have to do is think about that situation. See yourself in it.

(i) Whenever you feel under some stress, in a tight situation and perhaps feeling a sense of craving for a cigarette, create a space around you which contains all the details you have built up in your fantasy.

Normally, when you are under stress, relaxing is the very last thing you can do. However, by creating a space, you can consciously change the direction of your mental functioning. Your perception of the situation can become more objective. You allow your mind to stay in its non-smoking groove. Your mental functioning can remain more stable and calm and you won't trigger negative emotional responses which may put you in danger of being pushed out of your track. Remember, as soon as you feel that you are spiralling downwards into an emotionally tense state, create a space.

It is probably not part of your normal behaviour to suddenly stop what you are doing, and to close your eyes for a few moments. However, if you make yourself do it when you feel tense or if you feel like smoking a cigarette, you will keep yourself cool and calm, and in control of yourself.

Exercise

Taking a brisk walk or going for a short run is beneficial for your health, and many people find moderate exercise an excellent way of relieving tension and reducing the desire to smoke. Combine some exercise or activity with the other techniques you are already using. You will discover that you will begin to feel so much more healthy.

Breathing Away the Desire to Smoke

Deep breathing, combined with another awareness-heightening technique, taking your pulse, will relax you and change your awareness from the desire to smoke to concern about your health. Use this technique when the desire to smoke is very intense. Do not, however, use this technique in place of deprogramming. This technique should be reserved for near-crisis situations.

(a) Empty your lungs as completely as you can – this requires some effort. Now breathe in deeply and slowly.
(b) Hold your breath for a moment.

(c) Finally, breathe out fast. If possible, breathe out explosively, relaxing yourself fully.

(d) Now take your pulse. Your radial pulse point is on the inside of your wrist, just below the base of your thumb. Press your fingertips lightly to the pulse point, watch the second hand of a clock or watch, count the beats over the course of fifteen seconds, and multiply the result by four. Record your pulse rate. This will remind you of how healthy you are becoming as an ex-smoker.

(e) You should carry on breathing deeply while taking your pulse.

(f) Repeat the procedure, if necessary, then become occupied with something interesting. Involve yourself fully with that activity, as if it were the most important thing in the world.

Encouraging Words

We all respond well to encouragement. In this book you will find some encouraging thoughts, should you find yourself having to fight any battles. Remember, giving encouragement to others is also very strengthening. If you know someone else who is quitting smoking, phone them and encourage them to keep up the good work. Or phone a friend for a chat – they'll probably be pleased to hear from you.

It is also important to encourage yourself! There is a very simple, but useful technique which will help you stop generating negative thoughts. Your mind may generate thoughts such as: 'I'm no good, I'm a failure. I'll never do it. The others will stop, but I'll fail for sure. I can't do it. I'm weak. I've never been able to succeed. I'm hopeless.' When you become aware of the fact that your biocomputer is generating these thoughts, and flooding your mind with them, mentally shout the word, 'Stop!' Then deliberately start generating positive encouraging thoughts. You may like to use a Positive Programming Card. Write down some positive, encouraging statements on a card and keep the card with you. If you feel that you are becoming discouraged, take out your card and read it through. Here are some good examples:

- Each and every day I am getting better and better.
- I am losing the desire to smoke.
- I am a successful non-smoker.
- I am becoming healthy, free, and in control.

If your biocomputer then starts telling you again, 'But I really am weak,' repeat 'Stop!' and go back to the positive programming.

Remember, whether you feel weak or strong, a success or a failure, depends partly on what you tell yourself. Failures are often failures purely because they allow their biocomputers to generate negative failure-oriented thoughts. With such thoughts flooding their minds, how can they be anything other than failures? By consciously and deliberately repeating positive thoughts and statements, and passing them through your mind, your whole behaviour and attitude of mind will follow a much more positive and constructive direction. If you have a partner or friend who can also encourage you, so much the better. Ask them to encourage you as often as possible.

Distraction

If you are able to distract your mind from thinking about cigarettes for 60 seconds, your desire to smoke will pass the crisis point. To use a distraction technique, you simply focus on some problem which will keep your mind occupied for a short while. It may be necessary to really force yourself to get started but, once started, you will find that your mind becomes increasingly involved and the domination of your consciousness by the desire to smoke will fade. If you enjoy crosswords, have some handy. If you feel like smoking, take out a crossword and work on it for a few minutes. Keep a book of short stories or a novel handy. If you feel like a smoke, read a few pages. Select a book that you know will hold your interest.

Willpower

Many smokers have asked me this question: should willpower be used on D-Day? The answer is a resounding yes. At this point, you should find that you have enough confidence, assertiveness, and positive motivation to go full steam ahead, whatever happens, without smoking. If you have followed the procedures outlined, you should be able to manage this final stage by resisting any desire to smoke.

James' Progress

On Saturday, James smoked five cigarettes. On Sunday, he did not feel like going out and only smoked two cigarettes. He was feeling very pleased with himself. He planned setting a 'D-Day'. He used more of the visualization and implementation intentions techniques. James decided to make Tuesday his D-Day. He woke up on Tuesday, ready for the challenge not to smoke. He felt like a cigarette in the afternoon but resisted. He did not smoke from Sunday to Thursday. He found Thursday evening difficult but he used 'Create a Space' and went for a brisk walk, and then called into the pub for a drink with his friends. He refused to smoke. That was a major turning point. James resolved *never* to smoke again, and he never has!

Summary

- Keep active, relaxed, and reprogram constantly.
- Explore all of the different relaxation exercises at the weekend. Discover which ones work best for you and use them regularly from now on.
- Construct your very own Positive Programming Card. Use it every time you feel you need some encouragement. Your partner or friends should also be enlisted to support and encourage you.

- On D-Day itself, a little bit of willpower may be necessary. But by then you will have made excellent progress and you should be able to succeed.
- When you have completed your D-Day without smoking, you are half way to becoming a non-smoker.

How To Get a New Life as a Non-smoker

Part Three is designed for the quitter who has completed Part Two. To continue with Part Three, you need to cut your consumption to zero, and successfully complete your D-Day without having a puff of a cigarette.

If you have not yet completed a smoke-free D-Day, please work your way through Part Two again, setting yourself a new and *achievable* D-Day, until you have made it through the whole day without a single puff. Everything necessary is there. Please ensure that you follow the instructions in Part Two in every detail.

As soon as you have successfully completed your D-Day, return to this part of the book and learn how to maintain your new life as a non-smoker.

8

Preventing Lapses and Relapses

Now you are beginning your new life without nicotine. You are now able to give yourself a mega-amount of extra health, vitality and quality of life. You are on the way to becoming a brighter, calmer, cleaner, clearer, fresher, sharper, all-round healthier person. Your self-esteem will become stronger and your confidence will grow. Your non-smoking family members, friends, and colleagues will be breathing a huge sigh of relief. No longer will they have to put up with your addiction to tobacco. You are well on the road to recovery.

But all of these things can vanish as quickly as they came if you are not careful to monitor your experience and behaviour. You are still very vulnerable to smoking triggers. Think how long you spent smoking.

Deprogramming, reprogramming, eliminating triggers, reducing the desire to smoke, reducing your consumption of cigarettes and then stopping smoking for one day are all important steps in overcoming your smoking habit. For most smokers who quit for life, it's relatively easy to stop smoking for the first few days. However, they often start smoking again. You need to be absolutely committed to making the change permanent.

Smokers are often left to their own devices just after they stop smoking, and are given very little help. Yet this is the crucial stage where some informed guidance can make all of the difference. Quitting your smoking habit has involved many different processes: new skills, de- and reprogramming, relaxing, destressing, and a different self-image. At this stage, you need strategies for maintaining a smoke-free lifestyle for the rest of your life. You will need to use coping strategies when you're with other smokers, especially when they're your work colleagues, friends, or family members.

Part Three deals with the process of making your change permanent. Part Three will help you to:

- Learn how to prevent lapses and relapses.
- Be fully aware of the psychological factors that come into play when you have not smoked for an increasing interval of time.
- Learn new coping skills to help you deal with problems that may appear.
- Learn how to keep a check on your weight.
- Look at how you can increase your physical activity.
- Learn how to set up a new balance in your life in which smoking no longer plays a role.

The Diamond Stylus

A useful model of the ex-smoker has been described by two psychologists at the University of Washington, Alan Marlatt and Judith Gordon. They suggested that the smoker's life is like an old long-playing record spinning around on the turntable. A diamond needle moves along the spiral groove to produce sound from the record. The music flows from the beginning to the end, just like the smoker's life travels from the past to the present, and into the future. Ideally, what is needed is a smooth and continuous movement of the needle, with no disruption of its progress. However, occasionally, there may be an impediment along the groove of the record, causing the needle to jump. When the diamond needle of your life path jumps into the wrong groove, you lapse into the smoking habits of your past life. This not only spoils the music, it causes a disruption of the flow; you have to put the needle back where it belongs, and it isn't always easy to find the correct place on the record!

A life that flows smoothly is a joyful one. A life that is disrupted by an intrusive backslide is a miserable one.

When a smoking lapse occurs and the needle has jumped into the wrong groove, you are abruptly taken back into a previous stage of the record, repeating everything that has gone before. It's almost as if you never managed to give up smoking. And when it happens, you fear that it's going to repeat itself again and again.

Just as there are many forces that can make a needle jump out of its groove (e.g. dust, grease, scratches, cracks and breaks), so there are many factors which could knock you out of your non-smoking groove unless you are very careful – such as unexpected bad events, accidents, blows, bad luck and arguments, or when the stresses and strains of everyday living become intolerable.

Consider the following situation. Sandra has not smoked for five days. Today she has had a hard day at the office, with too much to do, and she has been working under a lot of pressure. This has led to a disagreement with her boss and her colleagues. Sandra comes home to find an unexpectedly high electricity bill waiting. She decides to use her credit card – until she checks the balance and discovers she's borrowed up to the limit. Sandra cooks dinner with her partner, Sam, and they share a bottle of wine. They relax after dinner in front of the TV. Sam lights a cigarette. Sandra experiences a compellingly forceful desire to smoke. After fighting it for a few minutes, she finally gives in and decides to have a cigarette.

This backslides Sandra right out of her non-smoking groove into her old groove of her life as a smoker. Now she is faced with the task of quitting smoking again. We can easily pinpoint a few of the forces that pulled Sandra so abruptly out of her groove:

- Stress during Sandra's day at work
- Sandra's physical addiction to nicotine
- Sandra's reprogramming not yet complete
- Alcohol acting as a trigger

- Sam's smoking acting as a trigger
- How many others?

Using CBT is giving you many advantages over someone as unprepared as Sandra. You have put into place psychological methods for removing your smoking programs and this type of lapse is therefore much less likely to occur.

However, there is still a danger that triggers will pop up which have not yet been permanently reprogrammed. Some of these may not have occurred during your last 7 to 10 days as a smoker, and therefore you will not have had a proper opportunity to reprogram them. You may also be suffering from the last stages of nicotine addiction, which may give you withdrawal symptoms and put you at risk of smoking again. There are solutions to these problems, but it will take more effort on your part. The next section gives further details about what you can do.

The Benefits of Quitting

It is useful now to assess what the benefits of quitting really are. Consider them in turn and then compile a full list of your own.

Rediscovered Senses

You may have noticed already how your senses of taste and smell have livened up. Many ex-smokers can't believe how tasty food really is, and how many scents they were unable to smell when they were smokers. You may find your appetite changes slightly, and foods or drinks which previously seemed bland become quite delicious. Some smokers worry that their new enthusiasm for eating will result in weight gain. A few pounds certainly may go on after stopping smoking, but you can just as easily take them off again, or at least limit the increase, by following the guidelines in Chapters nine and ten.

Cleanliness

You may notice the stench of stale smoke on your clothes. The smell of your hair and breath will improve greatly when you stop smoking. You may dislike the smell of smoke, and start to avoid social situations where smoking occurs. You will certainly feel fresher, brighter, and cleaner.

Physical Health and Fitness

Your health will improve as soon as you stop inhaling nicotine and carbon monoxide. These health improvements kick in at different times; the box on the following page gives more details. You may feel a lot more active, and you will be able to exercise for longer periods before you become tired. You could increase your level of physical activity by walking more, or taking more vigorous exercise such as running. If you are thinking of starting a more vigorous programme of exercise, it would be wise to consult your doctor first, to check the state of your heart and cardiovascular system. Follow the guidelines in Chapter ten.

Not everyone will experience all the changes listed in the box, especially people who lead sedentary lives or those who are already physically active. The long-term benefits of stopping smoking are considerable. Within a few years, your level of risk for smoking-related critical illnesses will fall to near-normal levels. A recent study found that the risk of lung cancer is reduced by 50 per cent in just five years after stopping smoking. Other evidence suggests that this reduction in risk kicks in even earlier.

Health Improvements After quitting Smoking

Within 20 minutes of your last cigarette:
- You stop polluting the air.
- Blood pressure drops to normal.
- Pulse rate drops to normal rate.
- Temperature of hands and feet increases to normal.

8 hours:
- Carbon monoxide level in blood drops to normal.
- Oxygen level in blood increases to normal.

24 hours:
- Chance of heart attack decreases.

48 hours:
- Nerve endings adjust to the absence of nicotine.
- Ability to smell and taste things is enhanced.

72 hours:
- Bronchial tubes relax, making breathing easier.
- Lung capacity increases.

2 weeks to 3 months:
- Circulation improves.
- Walking becomes easier.
- Lung function increases up to 30 per cent.

1 to 9 months:
- Coughing, sinus congestion, fatigue, and shortness of breath all decrease.
- Cilia (hair-like projections) regrow in lungs, increasing the ability of the lungs to handle mucus, clean the lungs, and reduce infection.
- Body's overall energy level increases.

1 year:
- Rate of death from heart disease is halfway back to that of a non-smoker.

5 years:
- Rate of death from disease is the same as that of a nonsmoker.

10 years:
- Rate of death from lung cancer drops almost to the rate of a non-smoker.
- Precancerous cells are replaced. The incidence of other cancers (such as: mouth, larynx, oesophagus, bladder, kidney, and pancreas) decreases.

Women's Health

Research shows that women benefit even more than men from quitting smoking. New findings from the 'Lung Health Study' in the US indicate that women's lung function improves significantly more than men's after sustained smoking cessation. The study followed more than 5,300 middle-aged smokers for five years. All participants had mild or moderate chronic obstructive pulmonary disease (COPD). In the first year after quitting smoking, the women's lung function improved more that twice that of the men's, although the differences between the genders narrowed over time.

Epidemiological studies have shown that menopause occurs between 0.8 and 1.7 years earlier in smokers than in non-smokers. Smoking can cause reduced fertility in women; in one study, smokers were more than three times more likely than non-smokers to have taken more than a year to conceive a child. It was estimated in this study that women who smoked were only 72 per cent as fertile as non-smokers. Smoking can also cause miscarriage. The Royal College of Physicians has suggested that there are 4,000 miscarriages a year in the UK caused by smoking.

Smoking during pregnancy carries significant risks for both mother and baby. The mother's airways function less well and may leave her physically unready for the birth process. The birth weight of the baby is also likely to be smaller and, as the baby grows, it is likely to remain shorter and lighter. This is because nicotine constricts your blood vessels, including the ones to the placenta and the baby, so the baby does not get enough oxygen and nutrients. However, the baby's health would be fine if the mother were to quit smoking about a month before trying to conceive. As we already discussed in Chapter one, you should have no nicotine at all in your system during pregnancy, since it constricts your blood vessels – including the ones to the placenta and the baby.

Sex

Many ex-smokers report that their interest in sex – and their actual sexual performance – increases after they quit smoking. This could be for several reasons. Firstly, they feel more attractive and more sexy. Secondly, the drug nicotine has a dulling effect on sexual appetite. Thirdly, the ex-smoker is more capable physically, runs out of breath less easily, and should be more sensitive to their partner's needs.

Several recent studies have looked at how smoking affects male impotence and found that there is a link between smoking and difficulties having an erection. Men who smoke are more likely to experience impotence and loss of stamina. Overall, smoking increases the risk of impotence by about 50 per cent for men in their thirties and forties. But the link between smoking and male impotence affects women as well. Nicotine is a vasoconstrictor, tightening blood vessels and restricting blood flow. In the long term, it causes permanent damage to arteries.

Since a man's erection depends on blood flow, it seems likely that smoking would affect erections. Studies have confirmed this. Forty per cent of men affected by impotence are smokers, as opposed to 28 per cent of the general male population.

It's difficult to say whether your sex life will definitely improve now that you have quit smoking, since many factors influence your sex life other than your ability to have an erection, but it certainly can help. Quitting smoking eliminates stained teeth, unhealthy skin, the rapid accumulation of wrinkles on the face, and the stink of smoke on your clothing, hair, and breath, which will make you more attractive to your partner.

Money, Money, Money

If health, fitness, and sex aren't enough to give you satisfaction, perhaps money will! A smoker burns up piles of money on cigarettes and this is money that they can usually ill-afford. You may be surprised to work out exactly how much you spend each year as a smoker. These figures will help with the calculation.

- Within two to five years, your risk of stroke is substantially reduced. You've also saved between £3,000 and £8,000.
- After 10 to 14 years, your risk of dying from cancer is nearly the same as that of a lifetime non-smoker. You've also saved over £17,000.
- After 15 years, your risk of coronary heart disease is nearly the same as that of a lifetime non-smoker. You've also saved over £25,000.
- At today's prices, if you smoke one pack of cigarettes per day for 10 years, you'll spend over £17,000 – easily enough to buy a new car.

Take time again now to calculate how much you used to spend per week on cigarettes. For every £1.00 a week spent on cigarettes during a working lifetime from the ages of 20 to 65, your cash outlay would be £2,340. If you invested this £1.00 a week at 5 per cent, the real cost would be £8,719. If you spend £20.00 a week on cigarettes, this figure would be £174,380. If your partner also smokes, that makes a total of more than a third of a million pounds gone up in smoke. Do you really want to spend so much on Cancer and Heart Disease LLC.

For Parents

One of the greatest benefits to parents who quit smoking must be the example that they set to their children. Your children are more likely to smoke if you are a smoker. A study published in 2000 carried out in Seattle, showed that parents who quit smoking before their child reaches third grade significantly reduce their child's chances of becoming a smoker by the time of their senior year of high school.

If one parent quits smoking by the time the child is 8 or 9 years old, the child's chances of being a daily or monthly smoker at age 17 or 18 decrease by 25 per cent. If both parents quit, the child's chances of smoking drop by nearly 40 per cent. If all smoking parents were to quit by the time their children were around age 8, this might be able to prevent 136,000 young people in the United States from becoming daily, long-term smokers, the Seattle researchers concluded.

It is likely that the same trends would be seen elsewhere. We model behaviour for our children. If they see us smoking, how can we expect them not to be tempted?

Self-Esteem

Other major benefits will be to your mental health, your sense of wellbeing, and your self-esteem. It is very difficult to feel good about yourself when you are trapped in a habit over which you have so little control. By ridding yourself of the habit, you will feel freer, more in control of yourself, and have higher self-esteem. This factor is often overlooked, but for many it is this increased sense of personal freedom, and all that this means, which makes stopping smoking worthwhile.

The World Health Organization has reported on the links between self-esteem, self-image and tobacco use. Adolescents who smoke tend to have low self-esteem, and low expectations for future achievement. They see smoking as a way to cope with the feelings of stress, anxiety and depression that stem from a lack of self-confidence. Any smoker who quits receives a helpful boost in self-esteem.

Personal List of Benefits Gained From Stopping Smoking Permanently

After considering the benefits listed above, give some thought to your own position. Write a list of your own personal benefits in the following table.

1 _____

2 _____

3 _____

4 _____

5 _____

6 _____

7 _____

8 _____

9 _____

10 _____

Think about these benefits and enjoy them. Mentally rehearse all of the desired outcomes of your new life as a permanent non-smoker.

Other Methods to Help You to Quit For Life

In this section I discuss the use of nicotine replacement therapy (NRT) in relation to Cognitive Behavior Therapy (CBT). Many people successfully use CBT or NRT as methods on their own. The combination of the two works better than either one alone. The US Department of Health and Human Services 2000 guidelines recommend that both behavioural and pharmacological treatments for smoking cessation are effective and should be combined. Health authorities generally claim that using nicotine patches doubles your chances of success. However, not everybody agrees. John R Polito claims that patches do not produce results any better than quitting on your own, and do far worse than intensive programmes such as CBT. However, we know that NRT helps to eliminate withdrawal symptoms. There are six main nicotine replacement products that can be considered:

- Nicotine gum
- Nicotine patches
- Nicotine inhaler
- Nicotine nasal spray
- Sublingual tablets
- Lozenges

These products vary according to speed of absorption, ease of use, frequency of use, type of side effects, and potential for the user to vary the dose to suit the needs of the moment.

Nicotine gum

Nicotine is the main factor in tobacco addiction. Within seven seconds of each puff of a cigarette, a high concentration of nicotine reaches the brain and changes the way it functions. It is this 'nicotine rush' that motivates smokers to continue the habit. Unfortunately no drug provides benefits only. Nicotine has both stimulant and sedative effects and, after it has been withdrawn from the body, unpleasant symptoms can develop, such as craving, irritability, difficulty in concentration, restlessness, and even bouts of depression.

Nicotine chewing gum is available from your local pharmacist without a prescription. Taken sensibly and in moderation, it can be an extremely useful aid at this stage. Although everything that can possibly be done to minimize withdrawal symptoms has been included in this programme (for example, meditation, relaxation and gradual reduction), it is still possible to experience withdrawal symptoms if your consumption was high or you had been a smoker for a very long time.

If you use nicotine products, it is essential to follow the manufacturer's directions. The gum should be used only when you feel the need for it during the first 10 to 30 days following D-Day. This will take the edge off any bad feelings that may result from stopping smoking.

Manufacturers recommend that you keep the gum in your cheek. You will then have it ready to chew on whenever you need it. Chew the gum only until you notice a slight tingling or peppery taste from the nicotine being released. Then keep the gum between your cheek and gum, so the nicotine can be absorbed. You should chew every 4 to 5 minutes for 30 minutes, until all the nicotine is released. You could use up to 30 pieces per day, for up to 6 months.

Hopefully your own usage will not need to be this high because you have already done a lot of deprogramming using the CBT. Nicotine gum comes in packs of different sizes. You may well require a relatively few number of pieces because your deprogramming and reprogramming will have achieved a lot in breaking your addiction to nicotine. Many CBT ex-smokers manage perfectly well with no gum at all.

Do not drink any hot liquids, tea or coffee, while the gum is in your mouth. Remove the gum, drink your beverage, and then re-insert the gum.

Always use the gum under medical supervision, especially if you have heart disease or are pregnant. Keep gum away from children and pets.

Different flavours are available, including spearmint, to disguise the bitter taste of nicotine and make the gum more palatable. A small minority of smokers have completely replaced the nicotine they obtained from smoking by chewing the gum! However this is not very likely, especially if you have already reduced your cigarette consumption to zero using this programme. The gum should be used as a very temporary bridge between smoking and non-smoking. It could therefore make all the difference in the first one to four weeks after stopping.

Some ex-smokers resist the idea of using the gum because they feel that they are replacing one kind of dependency by another. There are also possible side effects from the gum: sore jaw, mouth irritation, nausea, sore throat, heartburn, and rapid heart beat.

On the other hand, it is better to use the gum for a few weeks than to give in to the desire to smoke and lose everything that you have achieved so far. After a few weeks you will find that you can easily manage without the gum and you will then be free of nicotine forever.

Nicotine Patches

Another way of replacing nicotine is to use nicotine patches. These provide nicotine transdermally (through the skin) and have similar properties to nicotine gum, with the added advantage that the user can avoid the unpleasant taste. The patches help to abolish withdrawal symptoms, including irritability, tiredness and the craving to smoke. Patches give you a constant amount of nicotine in the bloodstream for the time the patch is attached. As far as nicotine is concerned, this means that there is a constant but small amount in your bloodstream. This should help to overcome the worst of the physical withdrawal effects, but they will not give the same effect or 'buzz' as inhaling on your cigarette.

There are different strengths of patches. The dosages are designed for smokers who are using patches and nothing else. Heavy smokers normally start on the highest strength, and work down to the lowest strength. Because you have been using CBT, you can probably skip the higher dose and start off with a moderate dosage, gradually reducing this to the lower dosage. There are a large number of possible side effects. The patches should not be used during pregnancy and breast-feeding or if you suffer from heart problems, stroke, or diseases of the skin. Your physician can advise you on the medical aspects of this form of nicotine. Please discuss the use of these with your doctor or pharmacist before starting to use them. Nicotine patches are available over the counter, but in the UK are also available from the National Health Service. Their prescription is linked to counselling in a local smoking cessation clinic.

Nicotine inhaler

The nicotine level from an inhaler peaks in 20 to 30 minutes. You can use the inhaler for upto 20 minutes every hour. About ten puffs on the inhalator is equivalent to one puff of a cigarette. It may cause coughing and throat irritation.

Nicotine nasal spray

This product gives the best relief from cravings. You can give one squirt to each nostril, once or twice per hour. It can be quite unpleasant at first, irritating your nose and throat, and it can make your nose runny. This product has the highest potential to recreate your dependence on nicotine so, in general, I do not recommend it.

Sublingual tablets

The 2 mg tablets dissolve under the tongue in 20 minutes, when the nicotine level peaks. Quitters normally have up to 30 tablets a day to replace cigarettes. However, your requirements, following CBT, could be much lower than this. The side effects are a stinging mouth, hiccoughs, and some gastric effects.

Lozenges

These come in 1, 2, or 4 mg doses and dissolve in the mouth in about 20 minutes. You move them around with your tongue every few seconds. As with sublingual tablets, the side effects are a stinging mouth, hiccoughs and gastric symptoms.

If you are still experiencing cravings, give these nicotine products serious consideration. A few days' or weeks' usage after your D-Day could make all the difference to your long-term ability to prevent relapse.

Social Skills for the Ex-smoker

The new non-smoking you will need skills and strategies to deal with the traps and pitfalls set by anybody who envies or resents the fact you no longer smoke, because they are still a smoker. This is one of the factors determining your long-term success or failure. Social pressure from smokers can sabotage your best efforts to quit.

Fortunately, you have a rich store of information about smoker psychology because, until very recently, you were one yourself!

A useful analogy is to think what it is like when, as a sober person, you deal with a person who is drunk: a fair degree of patience is needed because you are dealing with a person who cannot think logically or clearly, and whose befuddled mind is confused by splits in consciousness. You need to listen to what they say, but at the same time treat some of what is said with a large pinch of salt. In a friendly but firm manner, you will need to assert your right to choose not to smoke. Smokers will learn to accept this and respect you for making this decision.

Depending upon circumstances and how many smokers there are among your family, friends, and acquaintances, you will be exposed to a variety of opportunities to smoke. *You must never accept a cigarette when it is offered, nor weaken and ask for one.* You will need to practise being assertive while in the company of addicted smokers.

Many ex-smokers are struck by the selfishness of smokers almost immediately after stopping. This experience can be somewhat shaming as you realize how you yourself must have invaded other people's right to breathe clean, smokeless air over the period when you were a smoker. Therefore one of the biggest dangers for the new ex-smoker is to become rampantly anti-smoking. A tolerant, patient attitude is the best approach in the early days of non-smoking, no matter how secretly triumphant you feel on the inside.

The ex-smoker who quickly converts to being strongly anti-smoking probably still carries active Pro-Cigarette Programs

(PCPs) and is therefore still at risk. Deep down, some of the oldest, most stubborn PCPs are still partially active. Newer, non-smoking programs eventually override most PCPs. However, the fear that their deprogramming remains incomplete often motivates the most fervent anti-smoking evangelists. If you find yourself protesting to an extreme degree about other people smoking, you need to remain on your guard.

You probably have some deprogramming to do. Archaic triggers could remain partially hidden under cover of your consciousness. You must practise mental rehearsal at regular intervals to expel them. Choose the triggers that worry you the most and imagine yourself coping with them, even under severe provocation from others. By vividly imagining yourself happily dealing with these triggers, you will be able to supplant your PCPs with newer, more adaptive action programs. See yourself interacting with others, and smokers in particular, in ways that will minimize stress and conflict.

Continue to use relaxation in its various forms: meditating, fantasy, creating a space, and the other procedures described in Part 2. Continue to make time for these activities as a rite of passage.

Activity

You will find that you have more time on your hands as a result of stopping smoking. Many previous cigarette moments appear as gaps to be filled. Relaxation and other new activities are excellent ways of filling the vacuum.

Many people say that they do not know what to do with their hands when they give up smoking. That is unsurprising, when you think how much manual and oral activity goes into the behaviour of the regular smoker. You probably took 200 to 400 puffs of tobacco every day of your smoking life. There is the ritual of:

- taking out your cigarettes
- playing with one in your fingers
- lighting a match or lighter

- igniting the cigarette
- taking the first puff
- etc.

You were perhaps addicted to the ritual as much as to the nicotine. Many smokers also fiddle with their cigarettes or lighter while doing other things.

Some people find it helpful to play with a stress ball, a bunch of keys, or to doodle. Take up knitting, crosswords, or jigsaw puzzles – anything to keep your fingers busy for a few minutes until the desire to smoke passes. Some people take a sip of water or fruit juice every time they feel like smoking a cigarette. Doing a few push-ups or going for a run around the block can also help to relieve tension and keep your mind and body occupied when the desire for a cigarette becomes difficult to push away. The main thing is to keep your biocomputer busy with interesting things while mentally vacuuming, so that dormant PCPs can't keep popping out. There's nothing they like better than a passive, empty mind to fill! By now they should be seriously weakened, but if your mind is inactive something has to fill the vacuum.

Another option is to take up a few more physical activities. Full details about using physical activity for health and leisure can be found in Chapter ten.

The Fail-Safe Procedure

Now for the 'crunch' questions: what happens if everything suddenly fails? What will you do if, for some reason, you feel that you really *have* to smoke? What insurance policy do you have against that moment when you simply cannot resist smoking?

These are the questions that worry most ex-smokers, especially during the first few days after D-Day. They do have answers. There is an insurance policy. There is a fail-safe procedure. Although it is incredibly simple, it is one of the most crucial procedures in this entire programme. Use it if you ever feel that you cannot possibly avoid having a cigarette. Unfortunately, it is not very pleasant. However, it is far better to experience a few unpleasant minutes than to start smoking again, which will be what happens if you let yourself play the 'Just One' game. The Fail-Safe procedure is also called the 'Smoke Two Rule'. This is what you should do. Light a cigarette and smoke it. Then light a second cigarette and smoke, and smoke, until you feel so sick that you cannot smoke any more. You may need a third cigarette to really get smoking out of your system. However, if you do smoke until you are almost sick, you will not be at risk of developing the habit ever again. Experience with lapsing non-smokers has shown that the Fail-Safe Procedure is a successful prevention device. Use it, should you ever need to do so, at any time in the future. Your ability to remain a non-smoker forever is then a strong possibility.

Summary

- Make a list of the benefits that you personally will obtain from making non-smoking permanent.
- If you feel cravings for a cigarette, use a nicotine replacement product over the next few days and weeks.
- Learn social skills for dealing with smokers: be assertive, tolerant, and patient.
- Continue to use methods of relaxation.
- Keep your mind active – an empty mind is vulnerable to dormant PCPs that may spring back to life again if nothing else is keeping your mind occupied.
- If all else fails, use the Fail-Safe Procedure.
- Enjoy your first few weeks as an ex-smoker!

Managing Your Weight

One of the biggest fears many smokers have about quitting is that they will put on weight. You may have gained a pound or two already and you could be concerned about your waistline and looks. If so, do not despair. By using the techniques explained in this chapter, you can limit the extra weight you put on, and avoid any increases larger than is absolutely necessary.

There are hundreds of weight control and dieting systems available. Unfortunately the majority make bogus claims that can never be substantiated with any evidence. They appeal to the panic and desperation that can overtake a person who sees their weight escalating and running out of control. For example, I received the following spam email:

Hello, I have a special offer for you . . .
WANT TO LOSE WEIGHT?
The most powerful weight loss is now available without prescription . . .
100% Money Back Guarantee!
– Lose up to 19% Total Body Weight.
– Up to 300% more Weight Loss while dieting.
– Loss of 20–35% abdominal Fat.
– Reduction of 40–70% overall Fat under skin.
– Increase metabolic rate by 76.9% without Exercise.
– Boost your Confidence level and Self-esteem.

There are several features of this message that are somewhat difficult to believe. The figures seem spuriously precise – e.g. why 76.9% and not 76.8%? We cannot be sure whether such offers are going to be helpful to the recent quitter, because there is no evidence that a particular product would help you in this situation. Rather than relying on magical cures in the form of herbs, pills and potions, a much surer approach is to take the problem into your own hands by controlling your eating behaviour and increasing your levels of activity. The basic equation is as follows:

Energy stored as fat (Fat) = energy in (Food) – energy out (Exercise)

Or, simply,

FAT = FOOD MINUS EXERCISE

You can immediately see what you need to do if you want to lose weight. Eat less fatty foods and take more exercise.

Another worry for some people is that they will drink more alcohol when they give up smoking and risk becoming an alcoholic. One ex-smoker told me that he'd never had any real problems giving up smoking, although he confessed that alcohol 'helped'. I asked him how much he was drinking and he told me about a half-bottle of whisky every evening! However, substituting alcohol for smoking is not all that common, and the evidence suggests that smokers drink more than ex-smokers. A useful book for anyone whose drinking is causing them problems is *Let's Drink To Your Health* by Ian Robertson and Nick Heather. Although this is a less common worry, some ex-smokers definitely feel the need for something to replace their puffing on cigarettes.

Making some small but persistent adjustments to your eating or drinking habits, and to your present level of physical activity, are usually all that is required. You will find many different approaches to try here, and you should select methods that have the most appeal to you personally. As you work through this chapter, have a pencil handy so that you can write down your answers to the questions, and tick the relevant boxes when you come to a technique that you would like to try. Developing your new life as a non-smoker will take some time, as you will have many small adjustments to make. Gradual but successful improvements are what you should be aiming for, rather than radical, instantaneous solutions.

This chapter concentrates on eating because that is what usually causes most concern, but everything suggested can be applied equally well to drinking habits.

Are You a Healthy Weight?

Take a straight line across from your height (without shoes) and a line up from your weight (without clothes). Put a mark where the two lines meet.

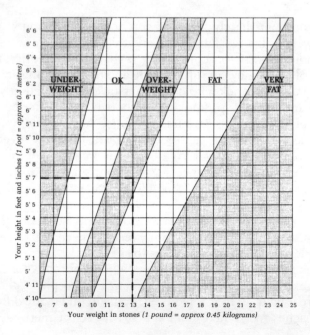

UNDERWEIGHT Maybe you need to eat a bit more. But go for well-balanced nutritious foods and don't just fill up on fatty and sugary foods. If you are very underweight, see your doctor about it.

OK You're eating the right quantity of food but you need to be sure that you're getting a healthy balance in your diet.

OVERWEIGHT You should try to lose weight.

FAT You need to lose weight.

VERY FAT You urgently need to lose weight. You would do well to see your doctor, who might refer you to a dietician.

A Few Key Questions

A good way of beginning to think about your eating habits is to answer the five questions below. Place a mark in the column which best describes your current eating behaviour:

	Never	Some-times	Very often
1. Since stopping smoking, have you noticed yourself eating more at meal times?	☐	☐	☐
How much more? A second helping? Any particular types of food? Please specify:			

_____

_____

2. Have you noticed yourself eating between meals more often than you did in the past?	☐	☐	☐
How much more often? What sorts of foods? Are these the same sorts of snacks or are they different from those you used to eat when you smoked?			

_____

_____

_____

3. Have you noticed yourself eating when in
the past you would have lit up a cigarette? ☐   ☐   ☐

At what sort of times? (Please specify)
_____
_____

4. Thinking back over the last week, have
you found yourself snacking while doing
the following?

   a) watching TV   ☐   ☐   ☐
   b) reading   ☐   ☐   ☐
   c) listening to the radio/music ☐   ☐   ☐
   d) sewing/knitting/writing   ☐   ☐   ☐
   e) cooking   ☐   ☐   ☐
   f) working   ☐   ☐   ☐
   g) shopping   ☐   ☐   ☐
   h) driving   ☐   ☐   ☐
   Other situations? (please specify)
   i) _____
   j) _____
   k) _____

5. Can you remember yourself eating in
situations where you were feeling any
of these emotions?

   a) angry   ☐   ☐   ☐
   b) worried   ☐   ☐   ☐
   c) sad   ☐   ☐   ☐
   d) lonely   ☐   ☐   ☐
   e) tired   ☐   ☐   ☐
   f) depressed   ☐   ☐   ☐
   g) nervous   ☐   ☐   ☐
   h) excited   ☐   ☐   ☐
   Other feelings? (Please specify)
   i) _____
   j) _____
   k) _____

Constructing Your Personal Eating CBT Programme

Using the ideas below, please select three of the many possible ways in which you can control your weight and use them for the next three weeks. When you can see that you have made some real progress, you should try some of the other possibilities during the weeks that follow.

There are many possibilities presented here. As you answer each question, really try to give an honest answer. This will allow you to develop a personal programme that suits you. You will not be able to do all of these things at once but, as you read about each one, consider it as if you were going to do it. When you have finished reading all of them, you will be able to choose the specific changes you would like to make and the methods you will use to make those changes. Think about each question carefully and then write the answers in the spaces provided.

1. Eating at Mealtimes

If you wanted to reduce the amount you eat at mealtimes by just a little, which specific food items can you imagine yourself leaving? If you choose fatty or sweet foods, then you will only have to reduce the amount you eat by just a little to eliminate a lot of calories. Write some of your initial ideas inside this box:

```
┌─────────────────────────────────────────────┐
│                                             │
│                                             │
│                                             │
└─────────────────────────────────────────────┘
```

2. Eating Between Meals

If you wanted to control snacking, or eating between meals, what do you think would be easier or more convenient to control? Tick the appropriate box.

How <u>often</u> you eat between meals   B ☐

or

The <u>amount</u> of food that you eat on each occasion   C ☐

or

The <u>fat content</u> of your snacks   D ☐

3. Substituting Eating for Smoking

Have you noticed yourself eating at times when in the past you would have lit up a cigarette? If so, write down one or two of those kinds of situations that you would like to control.

> E

> F

4. Trigger Situations

In question 4 of the Key questions above (page 142), did you tick any situations in the *Very Often* or *Sometimes* columns? If you did, which two would you most like to be able to control by not eating or over-eating? (If you ticked the *Never* column for all situations, please leave the two panels below blank).

> G

> H

5. *Trigger Emotions*

In question 5, did you tick any of the emotions in the *Very Often* or *Sometimes* columns? Which two would you most like to be able to handle without needing to eat something?

When I am feeling . . .	I

When I am feeling...	J

6. *Prioritize*

Look at your answers, A-J, and see if you still agree with them. Having made any corrections or adjustments, decide which are the most important to work on. Tick the three most important ones. Of these three, which would be easiest to control, which would be the most difficult to control, and which would be in between? Write the corresponding letter in each box below:

The easiest to control   [ ]

The second easiest to control   [ ]

The most difficult to control   [ ]

These three changes are the ones that you should concentrate on over the next three weeks. Start immediately with the easiest, the next easiest in three days time, and the most difficult in one week's time. Now that you have decided what your priorities are, study the next section to discover how to begin changing and modifying your eating behaviour.

The Techniques

Try the techniques corresponding to the three priorities you have selected. The more you enjoy using the techniques, the more successful they will be. As you work through this section, you will need a pencil. When you come across an idea which appeals to you, place a mark in the box. Later you will be able to quickly select the best techniques to try.

1. Reducing The Amount You Eat At Mealtimes

Having stopped smoking, you are able to prevent an increase in your weight by decreasing the quantity of food that you eat. This needs to be only a very small amount at each meal. The first thing you must *not* do is to try to force yourself to do things using willpower. When people focus on something they know they shouldn't really have, they end up wanting it all the more. There is a child in every adult, screaming to do everything it wants. If you constantly say to yourself things like, 'I'm on a diet. I'm depriving myself. That food looks really delicious,' it is very likely that you will build up a strong desire to eat more. Here is a set of guidelines that minimizes the need for willpower.

(i) Reduce the amount you eat by a small quantity at each meal. Don't deprive yourself of major quantities of enjoyable food by going on a crash diet, because that will never work – and you know it. How you think about what you are doing will affect how well you cope with it. Rather than thinking that you are depriving yourself, see yourself as confidently and surely developing your health by eating just a little less. [ ]

(ii) Use a smaller plate so that your portion seems larger than it really is. This helps to prevent overeating by reducing the amount you eat by just a little without actually noticing it. Research has shown that people who eat too much food find greater satisfaction when eating from a smaller plate, even when they themselves have measured the same amounts of food onto a larger and a smaller plate. This may be partially an illusion, but why not use it to your advantage? See if it works for you. [ ]

(iii) Slow down your eating. Overweight people usually eat too quickly. There is a time-lag between the stomach being full and the 'stop eating' signal arriving in the brain. This means that, if you eat quickly, the signal that you have had enough comes too late and you eat more than you really need. By slowing down your eating, you will actually eat less and yet feel perfectly satisfied. [ ]

You can slow down your eating using the following methods:

(A) Pay more attention to the taste, smell and texture of your food. Really concentrate on it. You will be able to eat more slowly, enjoy your food more and eat less. [ ]

(B) Put down your knife and fork more frequently, for example after every one to three mouthfuls. [ ]

(C) Count the number of mouthfuls you eat. Take a short rest period after a certain number (for example, after four mouthfuls). [ ]

(D) Put your knife and fork down and take a one- to two-minute break during the meal. [ ]

(E) Be the last person to finish each course of the meal. [ ]

By using these slowing down methods for a few days, you will be able to change the automatic habit of eating rapidly. Try to make a game of it so that your mind is occupied and you can enjoy trying to be last at finishing and the slowest eater at the table.

(iv) Leave a small amount of food on your plate every time you eat. This will help you break the bad habit of eating just because there is food in front of you, rather than because you really want it. [ ]

If you decide to reduce the amount of food you eat at meal times, practise the various techniques outlined above (and perhaps think of some others yourself) and use them every time you have a meal. These techniques will help you to gradually modify your behaviour.

2. Reducing Snacking

(i) Always eat three regular, planned meals a day. [ ]

(ii) Carry a card with you and mark down every time you eat between meals. This is exactly the same procedure that you used when you were reducing your smoking. Becoming aware of how frequently you eat between meals is an important step in taking control over your behaviour. You may be surprised at just how often you do have snacks. You should include everything you eat, such as biscuits, sweets, and crisps. By charting and monitoring your snacks, you will be able to reduce their frequency. [ ]

(iii) Devise some personal rules for snacking. One young ex-smoker began to consider herself a chocolate bar addict and often ate three or four at a time. Janet felt as strongly about having them as she used to feel about cigarettes. She eliminated her addiction by following these three eating rules:

1 She allowed herself to buy only one chocolate bar at a time. She could eat as many chocolate bars as she wanted but she could buy only one at a time.

2 She allowed herself to eat it in only one place – the cafeteria at her workplace.

3 She kept a reliable note of every one that she ate.

Knowing that she could have an unlimited number of chocolate bars took away her fear of deprivation but, by following the rules, Janet successfully eliminated her 'pro-chocolate programming' that made her constantly eat them. By recording her consumption and allowing herself to eat in only one place, she regained control over her behaviour. If she had tried to use willpower by stopping eating chocolate bars completely, you can imagine what would have happened. She would have quickly broken down and perhaps given up trying to control her eating behaviour completely.

(iv) Make up a set of your own personal rules for snacking con-
cerning when, where, and on what you are allowed to snack.
1 Decide exactly where you will allow yourself to snack,
and then only snack there. For example, you may decide
that you will snack only in the dining room at home,
and in the staff room at work. Whatever you decide,
write it down on the Progress Chart provided (see
Appendix C: Rules for Snacking).
2 Decide exactly when you will allow yourself to snack
(for example, only at particular times in the morning
and afternoon). Whatever you decide, write it down on
your Progress Chart.
3 Decide exactly what you will allow yourself to snack on.
Your aim should be to reduce the total number of calories you eat. You can change what you eat by choosing
only low-calorie snacks. If you normally eat two cookies
at morning coffee break, you may decide to eat just one
low-calorie cookie. Or you may decide to switch to a different kind of very low-calorie snack, such as raw celery,
cucumber, carrot, cauliflower, radishes, or fruit such as
oranges, plums, peaches, or apples.

It may seem useless to make such small changes to your
eating habits. However, given time, such little changes add up.
By making small adjustments now, you will avoid developing a
bigger weight problem later. Because they are only small adjustments to your eating behaviour, you should be able to incorp-
orate them more easily into your daily routine.

3. *Deprogramming Unwanted Eating Habits*

Just as having a cup of coffee sets off the desire to smoke in
many people, so different triggers can produce a desire to eat.
Obviously, you can't deprogram the desire to eat completely
but, when something triggers the desire to eat at an in-
appropriate moment, you should do something about it if you
want to have better control over your weight.

One woman realized that every time she walked past a candy shop, she got a strong desire to eat something sweet. Without even thinking about it, she would just walk in and buy some candy. A few moments beforehand, she had had no desire to eat candy; but, upon seeing the shop, she automatically went in and bought herself some. It didn't occur to her for over a year that the sight of the candy shop was a very potent trigger to eat candy.

To deprogram your snacking triggers you can use the same Three Steps (Stop – Think – Deprogram) which have proved so helpful in stopping smoking. Every time you feel a desire to eat outside one of your permitted times, you should:

1. STOP

2. THINK What is the trigger? What's making you feel like eating? Notice if something is happening which is triggering the idea that you would like to eat something. When you discover what it is:

3. START DEPROGRAMMING Tell yourself in a firm, forceful way what you will do next time that trigger appears. For example: 'Just because I'm walking past a shop that sells candy doesn't mean I have to eat candy. The next time I walk past a candy shop, I don't want to automatically feel like eating candy. The next time I walk past a candy shop, I won't automatically feel like eating. Don't send me those eating triggers. I'll choose when, where, and what I'll eat.'

The Three Steps should be used for every one of your snacking triggers which occur outside of your agreed eating times. You may find that some of them are really old smoking triggers. Treat them in exactly the same way. Write a list of triggers in your Progress Chart (see Appendix A). Once you have completed your deprogramming, you will find that you will be less likely to experience a strong desire to nibble or eat the next time you are in that situation. If you still feel the desire to eat something, don't deprive yourself, but follow the rules for snacking you have set yourself as to what and how much you are going to eat. Remember, each time you deprogram yourself and follow your new rules, you are gaining more and more control over your behaviour. Take it gently and, above all, enjoy doing it. The more you enjoy doing it, the more often you will use the techniques, and thus the greater control you'll have over your own behaviour.

4. *Alternative Scenarios For Trigger Emotions*

Many people have learned to cope with emotional situations by smoking or eating. For a compulsive smoker or eater, it is difficult to imagine not lighting up, or not going to the refrigerator when feeling fed up, angry or bored. Smoking or eating when in a bad mood doesn't actually solve the problem which triggered the emotion in the first place, even though smokers and compulsive eaters often think that it helps or that it is at least better than doing nothing. Unfortunately, in the long run, these unwanted habits can actually make you feel even worse.

A little time spent considering alternative behaviour beforehand can be of great value in avoiding eating or smoking when an emotional crisis occurs. Emotional upsets of one sort or another are inevitable for all of us, but it is also inevitable that they will pass away in time. And, when they have passed, it is very disappointing indeed to find yourself smoking again or a few pounds heavier. Look over the following list of alternatives. As you read them, try to think of something more appropriate to do. Write down your ideas as you explore possibilities. As you read through the list, mark off those suggestions which you find particularly appealing or which you at least feel are worth a try. Add ideas of your own.

When you are in the grip of a negative emotion or feeling, it is so easy to say: 'What the hell, I don't care any more. I feel so rotten, I don't care if I start smoking again, or if I do get fat.' That kind of helpless, hopeless thinking is precisely what keeps people eating too much food and may even bring about a relapse of smoking. When the crisis passes, as it always does, you will be very pleased that you have prepared an alternative scenario to help you cope while you are down. Change the scenario. Write yourself a new script. Be your own person. Do it now! Feeling worried, angry, sad, or lonely? When you are feeling any of these negative emotions, choose one of the following activities instead of eating, drinking, or smoking. Mark off any idea(s) which you would like to try. While you are doing so, also consider the need to increase your activity level.

(A) Something physical
  [ ] exercise, for example:

  _____

  [ ] weed the garden
  [ ] clean your house, or
  [ ] _____
  Physical exercise could have lots of positive benefits over and above helping keep your weight down; see Chapter nine for further details.

(B) Use a relaxation technique for 20 minutes or so.
  [ ] relax to a record you like
  [ ] meditate for 20 minutes (as your mind returns to thinking about your problems, gently go back to your mantra)
  [ ] take a hot, relaxing bath, or
  [ ] _____
  You may be surprised what a difference a little relaxation can make to the way you feel.

(C) Deliberately divert your attention from your feelings by imagining something pleasurable.
  [ ] think about a book you like
  [ ] think about a movie you saw recently and enjoyed
  [ ] think about a friend you particularly like
  [ ] think about an outing you enjoyed or

  _____

  [ ] _____
  A technique like this may not solve your problem, but it helps to take the pressure off, helping you to be more rational, and less likely to eat or smoke.

(D) Do something pleasurable.
  [ ] read a book

[ ] watch TV, a DVD or video
[ ] visit or phone a friend you like
[ ] go for a walk in the park
[ ] involve yourself in a hobby or .
[ ] _____

When you feel bad, remember that it takes a conscious decision to deliberately make the effort to do one of these activities. It is easy to say to yourself: 'Reading won't do any good. It won't help the situation.' But remember that doing this is not intended to solve the problem; it will give you time out so you can handle the situation better.

(E) If your worry is caused by a specific problem, try to talk it over with a supportive person, rather than simply do nothing other than eat or smoke.

5. *Mentally Rehearse Your New Eating Behaviours*

Having successfully stopped smoking, you have set in motion a number of different processes in your body and started a healthier lifestyle. Having got this far, it would be a great pity to lose any of the achievements you have made, and for this reason you should continue to use your imagination creatively. In your imagination, your thoughts, images and ideas can gain control over your behaviour and your new life can develop. Your imagery provides a powerful method of practising new activities, ways of coping, and changes in lifestyle.

When you settle down at night, ready for sleep, and begin to relax, this is a perfect time to work with your imagination. In the few minutes just before you drop off to sleep, think about what you have done during the day. Think of the things you have done with which you aren't entirely satisfied. Imagine how things might have been. By imagining yourself acting, behaving, eating, or drinking differently, you set into motion the very processes that will begin to change your behaviour. For example, you may remember that you felt hassled at work. Other people were bothering you and not letting you get on with what you really wanted to do. Almost automatically, your mind flashed on your cigarettes. Even now your old PCPs are lying dormant, still not completely eliminated. You went out and got yourself a packet of peppermints and ate the whole bag during the course of the afternoon, hardly in line with keeping your weight down.

As you lie in bed relaxing, think about the situation again. But this time imagine acting in a quite different manner. You might see yourself expressing your irritation directly to whoever it was that upset you. This is much more adaptive than going out to buy those peppermints. Or you might choose to see yourself taking a deep breath, and imagine yourself eliminating the anger as you breathe out. See yourself doing this several times until, in your imagination, you can see yourself feeling calm again. Let your images do the work for you, by making them as real as possible. You can also use this time just before falling asleep to practise those techniques you have decided to use to control your eating. For example, if you have decided to leave a little food on your plate at every meal, imagine actually doing this. Imagine putting your knife and fork down, yet leaving a little food on the plate. You can prepare yourself and get used to the idea that you don't have to eat everything. Imagine that this has become a quite normal and regular thing to do. Anticipate the comments your family might make and how you would explain to them what you are doing.

By choosing what to do in your imagination, you can begin to train your mind. Remember that there is always an alternative to eating, drinking, and smoking in response to negative emotions. By imagining yourself acting in new ways, you are actually writing new programs into your biocomputer. Your images provide new action plans and new models for your behaviour. By deliberately building new 'memories' of yourself acting differently, you will be surprised to find yourself acting in new ways, more or less automatically and spontaneously. If you mentally practise doing some exercise instead of going to the refrigerator when you feel sad, you will find that the next time you do feel sad, the chances of actually doing some exercise, rather than eating, will be greater.

The principal guideline is to make any change in your behaviour slowly and gradually. Although your imagery might be quite powerful, and make you feel capable of managing almost anything, don't demand too much at any one time and don't try to see yourself making dramatic changes overnight. Do not try to reprogram yourself with things like: 'From tomorrow onwards I will not eat between meals,' because it simply won't be possible that quickly. If you eat between meals very often, you will end up being disappointed when you fail to maintain your decision every single time a trigger appears.

Willpower is no more useful now than it was giving up smoking. Imagine yourself changing gradually, slowly getting better and better, changing your behaviour systematically and surely, rather than doing it all in a rush and being defeated.

Let's consider this example. Since stopping smoking, suppose that you have developed the habit of eating peppermints all day. Instead of cutting them out all at once, use mental rehearsal to imagine eating them only at certain times, or making a packet last two days instead of one. By making slow changes, and nothing too dramatic, you are more likely to succeed progressively, until you find you are eating peppermints only occasionally. By cutting them out all at once, you increase your chances of failing, becoming discouraged and then not bothering to try any more. You can achieve remarkable things if you use your imagination to plan action in a systematic fashion.

Summary

- The same methods that helped you to stop smoking can be applied to your eating and drinking, if they become a problem.
- Your weight can be controlled in two ways: by reducing your consumption of fattening food and by increasing your bodily activity. By eating healthier food and taking more exercise, your weight will normalize.

- Go through the targets A-J listed in the chapter and set yourself three priorities. Work towards achieving these targets, one after the other.
- Select those methods that you find most useful or appealing personally. Small changes made slowly are more successful than large changes made quickly.
- Use imagery rehearsal and the Three Steps to reduce snacking between meals and to change your eating habits.
- Whatever else you do, remember that smoking is a thing of the past. Take one day at a time and your weight can be slowly but surely restored to its pre-quit level.
- Continue to enhance your general wellbeing and enjoyment of life by maintaining your programme of relaxation.

10

Becoming More Active

When smokers quit, a major change occurs in the pattern of their activity. A typical 25-a-day smoker takes around 100,000 puffs per year from over 9,000 cigarettes. The total time taken up by smoking is the equivalent of one whole month out of every year. Smokers also tend to take less physical exercise than non-smokers. Stopping smoking therefore creates an 'activity gap' and a 'time gap' which need to be filled. This chapter contains guidelines on how these gaps can be filled by incorporating new activities into your lifestyle.

For many people, neither problem will be all that serious. Other things, for which there hadn't previously been enough time, simply fill the gap left by smoking. Smoking is something that is rarely done on its own. However, for those who smoked a lot of the time while alone, there will be a highly noticeable gap to fill. It is for this group that this chapter will be especially useful. Increased physical activity can benefit anybody looking for ideas to improve their general wellbeing.

The 'Fidget Factor'

Smokers fall into two types – those for whom the effects of nicotine are most important, and those who see smoking as an important way of filling gaps in their daily activities. When people in the latter group quit smoking, they need to have something else to do with their hands and also possibly their mouths. Activities such as fidgeting, doodling, tapping or twiddling small objects may all be useful especially during the first few weeks. You could buy a special 'stress ball', made of soft foam rubber, to keep in your hand or a pocket; a squash ball would serve the same purpose. It's quieter than playing with a bunch of keys, which may irritate others. Worry beads may also provide a useful substitute.

Substitute oral activities which have proved helpful for new non-smokers include chewing gum, sipping fruit juice or water, and gritting your teeth. Some ex-smokers feel fidgety and restless and constantly move or jiggle about. If you find yourself with this restless feeling, you'll probably find yourself automatically doing one or more of the activities listed above. Your restlessness will eventually die down to tolerable levels. There are also ways your new energies can be channelled into beneficial activities and physical exercise.

Physical Exercise

Most people take far less exercise than is desirable from a health point of view. The passive viewing of TV has taken over as the dominant form of social and recreational activity. The couch potato who stops smoking is therefore more likely to experience the restless, empty feeling than those who are physically active, and will need to avoid eating to fill the gap (see Chapter nine for more details). It's also a good idea to consider starting an exercise plan.

Regular exercise enhances a positive mood, reduces depression and anxiety, and generally leads to increased wellbeing. A personal exercise programme will help you to fill the activity gap, if you experience one, and will also raise your general level of fitness. All these factors provide a clear bonus for your physical health.

Exercise: Why Bother?

- Exercise helps you feel good.
- It's great fun, and a good way of making new friends and enjoying your leisure time more.
- It helps you feel more energetic.
- It helps you relax.
- It helps you get slim and stay slim.
- It helps keep you supple, and also more mobile as you get older.
- It helps strengthen your muscles, joints, and even your bones.
- It helps your heart work more efficiently and improves your circulation
- It needn't cost anything.
- The more you do, the easier it becomes.

What is Fitness?

Suppleness

This means being able to bend, stretch, twist and turn through a full range of movement. You need it for awkward jobs around the house, and getting in and out of different forms of transportation, If you're supple, you're less likely to get injured and you'll be able to stay more active as you get older.

Strength

This means being able to exert force – you can can push, pull and lift. You need strength to move around, carry shopping bags, climb upstairs, and take stubborn tops off bottles! Strength protects your body from sprains and strains. A strong back and stomach will improve your posture, too.

Stamina

This means being able to keep going, when running or walking briskly, without getting tired or out of breath very quickly. Stamina is useful when you're in a hurry to get somewhere, or when you need to keep up with your children! Exercising for stamina helps to protect you against heart disease. The best activities for stamina are are those which are more energetic than you are used to doing, make you slightly out of breath and keep you moving for 20 minutes or more. This type of exercise is often called 'aerobic' exercise, because it makes you breathe in enough oxygen to supply your working muscles. Lots of the activities in this chapter fall into this group.

Are You Willing to Exercise?

There are a lot of excuses you could use to avoid exercise – but they're very easily answered.

'It's too much hard work. I'd never keep it up.' It won't seem like hard work if you choose an exercise you enjoy and build up the length of exercise time and intensity slowly and gradually. As you get better, you'll enjoy it even more and you won't want to give it up.

'I haven't got time. My life is too busy.' Just 20 minutes, two or three times a week, can keep you active. Once you start feeling the benefits, and your new activity becomes a habit, it'll be easy to put aside the time.

'What I need is relaxation.' Exercise can be just the thing to help you relax. It relieves stress by talking your mind off your problems. After a session of vigorous exercise, you'll feel warm, comfortable and relaxed. You'll notice the relaxing effect of some kinds of exercise even while you're doing them. Recent studies have shown that exercising can also lift depression. You'll probably find it helps you sleep better, too.

'But doesn't it have to hurt to do you any good?' No. If it hurts, then you're pushing yourself too hard. If you're in any pain, stop immediately. If you feel uncomfortably out of breath, slow down.

'It's too late for me – I'm past it!' It's never too late. Anyone can get fitter. Whatever your age, you can find a form of exercise that will suit you. The less fit you are to start with, the sooner you'll notice the benefits.

'But isn't it bad for my heart?' On the contrary, it helps to protect your heart. When you exercise, your muscles need more oxygen than usual, so your heart has to beat faster to pump more oxygen-carrying blood to them. If you exercise regularly, your muscles get better at using oxygen and your heart pumps more blood with each beat, so it doesn't need to beat so fast. As you get fitter, you can exercise harder without overtaxing your heart. *Regular* exercise has other benefits too. It can help to control high blood pressure. It can also help stop your arteries furring up. Over the years, your risk of having a heart attack will be reduced.

'I'm not the sporty type.' Even if you didn't like sports at school, there are now so many different activities, you are sure to be able to find one you enjoy. Just try different ones until you find the one that's right for you.

'I couldn't do it on my own.' You don't have to. Clubs and classes are really good places to make friends, and lots of them have social events as well as exercise. Why not show this chapter to your friends and get them to go along with you?

'I'd be too embarrassed.' Don't let embarrassment put you off exercise – you'd be missing out on too much. People of all shapes and sizes enjoy exercising, and you won't feel uncomfortable or out of place if you choose an activity that's right for you.

'I couldn't bear all the sprains and strains.' You'll only get these if you push yourself too hard, too soon, or if you do occasional sessions of hard exercise and nothing in between. If you start off gently and build up slowly, your risk of developing a sprain or strain is very low. Exercise also builds up strong muscles, which protect you from injury. When muscles aren't used, for example when a broken leg is put in a cast, the muscles waste away and the leg gets thin and weak. When muscles are used more than usual, for example while exercising, they get stronger and more efficient.

'I've got young children to look after.' It might take a bit more organizing, but it doesn't have to stop you exercising. Some sports centres have child-care facilities. Your local library should be able to tell you about facilities. Or you could get together with a group of other people with young children and share the baby-sitting.

'If I can't do it properly, then what's the point of doing it at all?' You don't have to go into serious training and get super-fit, or play competitive sports, to benefit from exercise. Regular activity for just 20 or 30 minutes, two or three times a week, will go a long way towards helping you stay in good shape.

'I'm too fat for that kind of thing.' Then you are just the sort of person who will benefit most from some regular exercise, especially if it's the stamina-building type. Most people don't need a medical check-up before starting to exercise. Exercising helps you get slim and stay slim by burning calories. If you burn more calories than you eat, your body will start using its own energy stores and fat will start to disappear. There's evidence that some people may still be burning up more calories than usual after they have finished exercising – sometimes for several hours.

Before You Start

Sensible precautions

As long as you choose the right form of exercise, begin gently and increase the length and intensity of your exercise session gradually, you'll gain all the benefits without straining yourself. Always warm up first, with a few gentle bends and stretches, and cool down afterwards by walking slowly for a few minutes. Most injuries are caused by overuse of joints and muscles, so don't overdo it. In general, don't do anything vigorous unless you have built up to that level of intensity and you do it regularly.

Always ask your doctor about the best form of exercise for you if:

- You've had chest pains, high blood pressure or heart disease.
- You have chest trouble, such as asthma or bronchitis.
- You have back trouble or have had a slipped disc.
- You have joint pains or arthritis.
- You have diabetes.
- You're recovering from an illness or operation.
- You're worried that exercise may affect any other aspects of your health.

For all these conditions, exercise can be helpful, but it is a good idea to talk it over with your doctor first.

If you are over the age of 35, you should have your blood pressure checked by your doctor or at a clinic at least once every five years, whether or not you intend to take up exercise.

Having a disability doesn't mean you shouldn't exercise. You may benefit from regular exercise of the right kind.

If you're pregnant, there's no reason why you shouldn't continue with any sport or activity you already enjoy. Exercising in pregnancy is beneficial as long as you feel comfortable. However, do not start new exercise programmes when you're pregnant.

If you have a cold, a temperature or a sore throat, don't exercise until you feel better, and remember to start gradually again when you get back to exercising. Don't do any vigorous exercise for at least an hour after a meal.

Stop exercising immediately if you have any of these symptoms:

- pain
- dizziness
- feeling sick or unwell
- unusual fatigue

If the symptoms persist or come back later, or if you are worried about them, see your doctor.

Clothes and footwear

For most activities, you won't need to buy anything new. Just wear loose, comfortable clothes and a good strong pair of shoes.

For any activity which involves a lot of running or jumping you will need a good pair of running shoes to protect your feet, joints and back from damage. Make sure the shoes you buy have a thick, cushioned sole, especially at the heel, to prevent jarring of your joints. Check that the sole is wide enough for comfort, with plenty of room for your toes. Look for shoes with a good arch support and strong heel cup; this will stop your foot tilting inwards while you're running.

Remember you may need a size larger than your normal shoes, because your feet are likely to spread a little when you exercise, and you may be wearing thick socks.

Getting Started

If you're not very active now, your first step to getting fitter is simply to walk more. Why stand at a bus stop or sit in a traffic jam when, with a bit of effort, you can walk or bicycle the journey, or part of it, almost as quickly?

When you walk, walk faster. Walking briskly for 20 to 30 minutes, two or three times a week, will soon build up your stamina.

Use the stairs instead of the elevator, and walk up escalators. Climbing stairs is a good way of keeping your leg muscles strong.

Even if you are active at home, or at work, you'll probably still need other activities to give you enough suppleness, strength and stamina.

You'll find activities listed below which will give you a good balance.

Four Golden Rules Of Exercise

Get moving

Use more effort than usual by finding a more active way to do the things you usually do, and by taking up completely new activities. Move through a wider range of movements and keep going for longer.

Build up gradually

It takes time to get fit. Work hard enough to make yourself a bit sweaty and out of breath, but not uncomfortably so. That way, there will also be a lower risk of sprains and strains. Always warm up first, with a few gentle bends and stretches, and cool down afterwards by walking slowly for a few minutes.

Exercise regularly

It'll take 20 to 30 minutes of exercise two or three times a week for you to get fit and stay fit.

Keep it up

You can't store fitness.

Activities

There are hundreds of activities to choose from. Choose activities:-

- Which you enjoy.
- Which make you feel good.

- Which you can do regularly – for 20 or 30 minutes, two or three times a week.
- Which you can fit easily into your everyday routine, so there's no excuse for not keeping them up.
- Which you can do near home, so you don't have to travel far.
- Which don't depend on the weather or seasons.
- Which suit your particular fitness needs.

Here are some ideas to choose from:

- Walking
- Swimming
- Bicycling
- Jogging and running
- Golf
- Bowling
- Badminton
- Tennis
- Squash or racquetball
- Team Games
- Weight training
- Martial arts and judo
- Exercise classes
- Dance
- Yoga
- Exercising at home

Summary

- Get fit and stay fit! Once you're fit, you need to make sure you stay fit. Once you start becoming a naturally active person, staying fit won't seem difficult.
- The way to get fitter is to be more active and vigorous than you usually are.
- Try to choose the active ways of doing daily tasks, instead of the lazy ways. You'll be surprised what a difference small changes can make to your fitness.

- Choose a form of exercise you enjoy enough to do regularly, for at least 20 to 30 minutes two or three times a week, and make a habit of it.
- Whatever you choose to do, start gently and build up gradually. You don't have to strain yourself to feel the benefits of exercise.
- You don't have to choose just one thing. Try lots of different activities, to give you a good balance of suppleness, strength and stamina. Have fun!

11

Resisting Cigarette Marketing

In this chapter we will examine some facts and fallacies about tobacco marketing. Gradually tobacco advertising in its traditional form is disappearing. But it is being replaced by more subtle forms of marketing which has three main goals: to induce people to smoke; to induce existing smokers to switch brands; and to keep existing smokers loyal to the brand they already smoke. There is incredibly fierce competition between companies as they fight to retain their share of an ever-declining market in domestic sales but a fast-increasing global market.

The marketing strategies vary from country to country. For example, Wal-Mart is aggressively pushing Marlboro cigarettes in Latin America and Asia at supermarket check-out points, while refraining from the practice in the US. Apparently, the perceived value of life differs according to which side of the US border one lives! Looking at the issue purely statistically, the tobacco industry loses almost 5,000 customers every day in the US alone – 3,500 quitters and about 1,200 smokers who die. The most promising 'replacement smokers' are young people: 90 per cent of smokers begin before they're 21, and 60 per cent before they're 14. To find their new customers, every day US tobacco companies spend $11 million to advertise and promote cigarettes. This is more than the US Federal Office on Smoking and Health spends to prevent smoking in an entire year.

US youths are the biggest new customers for tobacco products. Cigarette advertising links smoking with being 'cool', taking risks, and growing up. At the same time, the tobacco industry insists that it does not want children to smoke – and backs up its claims with campaigns supposedly designed to discourage young people from smoking. But programmes such as 'Tobacco: Helping Young People Say No' are not only slick public relations efforts designed to bolster industry credibility, they actually *encourage* tobacco use among young people. By leaving out the health dangers, ignoring addiction, and glamorizing smoking as an 'adult custom', these campaigns reinforce the industry's advertising theme, presenting smoking as a way for children to exert independence and be grown up.

Internationally, cigarettes are marketed as a 'passport to prosperity'. Images of America and London are used to promote the idea that by smoking a USA or UK brand you can actually increase your chances of being transported there. The key messages are wealth, health, consumption – in other words, 'the US'. In developing markets from Eastern Europe to South-east Asia, trans-national tobacco companies hawk cigarettes using slogans such as 'L & M: The Way America Tastes', 'Winston: The Spirit of the USA' and 'Lucky Strikes: An American Original'. These themes and images expand the appeal of cigarettes to young people and women.

The tobacco industry has a unique problem: it is the only industry that actually kills off its longest-serving and most loyal customers! In the UK alone, between three and four hundred customers die every day as a result of smoking. Other people, like you, stop smoking and become lost customers. Tobacco companies are therefore constantly in search of new customers to replace those who die or quit.

Naturally, tobacco companies deny that their advertisements are designed to persuade young non-smokers to start the habit, but obviously they must find new customers if they are to stay in business. Research on smoking prevalence among young people suggests that the tobacco industry is rather successful in promoting smoking among young people. Children who are not yet smokers but who say that they approve of cigarette advertising are also twice as likely to start smoking. Research shows that children definitely are recruited to smoking.

In changing tobacco law, smaller countries have taken the lead in reducing levels of smoking. Norway, Iceland, and New Zealand all provide good examples of what happens when advertising is successfully banned. In 1975, 17 per cent of 13- to 15-year-olds in Norway were regular smokers when a complete ban on tobacco advertising was introduced. There has since been a steady drop and, by 1990, only 10 per cent of this age group in Norway were smokers. France, Italy, and Portugal also operate an advertising ban.

In 1971, the US Surgeon General proposed a government ban on smoking in public places. That year, cigarette advertising ended on radio and television and the cigarette manufacturers' voluntary agreement to list tar and nicotine yield in all advertising became effective.

Many countries have banned tobacco advertising and promotion. In 1998, the European Union adopted a directive to ban most tobacco advertising and sponsorship by July 30, 2006. Other countries have banned direct advertising, while others have brought in partial restraints. Such bans are often got around by tobacco companies through clever promotional ideas, such as retail stores named after cigarette brands, or corporate sponsorship of sporting events. National bans on tobacco advertisements may be rendered ineffective by tobacco promotion on satellite television, by cable broadcasting, or via the Internet.

The tobacco industry, and newspaper publishers who gain revenue from advertising, are a powerful lobbying group with a vested interest in preventing restrictive legislation. A leading article in *The Independent* (London) on 17 January 1992 typifies the wobbly thinking of the pro-advertising lobby:

From the health point of view, tobacco is the most dangerous consumer product on the market, causing an estimated 110,000 premature deaths a year in the UK . . . public smoking is anti-social, if not actually injurious to the health of those obliged to indulge in passive smoking. Heavy smokers smell disgusting, their smoke pollutes the clothes, hair and food of non-smokers in pubs and restaurants and at parties, creates litter and is a major fire hazard. The cigarette industry's claim that advertising does not increase overall consumption, but simply persuades smokers to switch brands, is ridiculous. Advertising increases the market for all other goods. Cigarettes are hardly likely to be an exception.

None the less, this newspaper does not support the Commission's proposed ban . . . As long as cigarettes are legal, it is illogical as well as illiberal to ban advertisements.

In spite of its self-proclaimed desire to be logical, the newspaper fails to reach the most logical conclusion of all: that, in the light of the facts so elegantly outlined in the above editorial, advertising *and* cigarette sales should be banned. That would also be seen as illiberal, an infringement on rights. After all, the government shouldn't try to prevent millions of people from dying a painful, premature death caused by smoking, if that is what they choose to do, should it?

Advertising Cigarette Smoking To Women

The Surgeon General produced a review of smoking among women in 2001, discussing the role played by tobacco advertising. Such advertising first became geared towards women in the 1920s. By the mid-1930s, cigarette advertisements aimed at women were so common that an ad for the mentholated Spud brand said 'To read the advertisements these days, a fellow'd think the pretty girls do all the smoking'.

Cigarette advertising for women has been oriented towards promotion of slimness, glamour and attractiveness. Messages such as 'Reach for a Lucky instead of candy' tried to establish an association between smoking and slimness. The positioning of Lucky Strike as an aid to weight control led to a greater than 300 per cent increase in sales for this brand in the first year of the advertising campaign.

Throughout World War II, Chesterfield advertisements featured glamour photographs of a Chesterfield girl of the month, usually a fashion model or a Hollywood star such as Rita Hayworth, Rosalind Russell, or Betty Grable.

Jean Kilbourne and Rick Pollay, in their 1992 book *Pack of Lies*, discuss the fact that, when smoking first came into vogue, it was considered a man's activity, a very unfeminine thing to do. Therefore it became a vehicle for women's rebellion and for asserting a new, more independent, self-image. Tobacco companies capitalized on this. A public relations expert, Edward Bernays, was hired by the tobacco industry. Women dressed like feminists were hired to march in the Easter Parade of 1929 in New York City. They were paid to smoke and the press referred to their cigarettes as 'torches of freedom'. This began an association between women smokers and freedom or liberation, and the tobacco industry has promoted that assocation.

The number of women aged between 18 and 25 who began smoking increased significantly in the mid-1920s, when the tobacco industry mounted the Chesterfield and Lucky Strike campaigns directed at women. The trend was most striking among women aged between 18 and 21. The number of women in this age group who began smoking tripled between 1911 and 1925, and had more than tripled again by 1939.

In 1968, Philip Morris' ads for Virginia Slims acknowledged the importance of the emerging women's movement with the slogan 'You've come a long way, Baby', later giving way to 'It's a woman thing' in the mid-1990s. More recently, the 'Find your voice' campaign has featured women of diverse racial and ethnic backgrounds. The underlying message has been that smoking plays a part in women's freedom, emancipation, and empowerment.

The Surgeon General found that initiation rates among girls aged between 14 and 17 years rapidly increased in parallel with the combined sales of the leading women's-niche brands (Virginia Slims, Silva Thins, and Eve). In 1960, about 10 per cent of all cigarette advertisements appeared in popular women's magazines and, by 1985, cigarette advertisements had increased by 34 per cent.

In current marketing strategies, women have been extensively targeted. This gender-specific marketing is dominated by themes of social desirability and independence, and smoking messages feature slim, attractive, and athletic models. In 1999, expenditure on domestic cigarette advertising and promotion in the US was $8.24 billion a 22.3 per cent increase from the $6.73 billion spent in 1998.

Advertising is intended to reduce women's fear of the health risks from smoking by presenting information on nicotine and tar content or by using positive images e.g., models engaged in exercise or pictures of white-capped mountains against a background of clear blue skies. However, cigarette brands developed exclusively for women (e.g., Virginia Slims, Eve, Misty, and Capri) account for only 5 to 10 per cent of the cigarette market. Many women are also attracted to brands that appear gender neutral or overtly targeted to males.

In the six years following the introduction of Virginia Slims cigarettes, the number of American teenage girls who smoked more than doubled.

All the companies need to do to escape legislation restrictions is to look for loopholes and then use them. Anything which they can do to link a brand name or image with a worthy-sounding cause helps to promote that brand. The tobacco industry has targeted the female market through corporate sponsorships. For example, in Canada the Matinee Ltd Fashion Foundation sponsors fashion designers. To escape advertising restrictions in Canada, RJR-Macdonald is using female celebrities to promote its Vantage brand by 'sponsoring' the 'Vantage Women of Originality Awards' in Canadian magazines. The women who receive these awards (Jann Arden and Holly Cole, for example) receive a profile in a major women's magazine, and a donation of $5,000 to a women's charity of their choice.

Not surprisingly, women's magazines that accept tobacco advertising are much less likely to publish articles criticising smoking than are magazines that do not accept tobacco advertising. Tobacco advertising tends to promote a culture of passive acceptance rather than active criticism of tobacco products. A study of women's magazines in Europe in 1996 to

1997 found that over half of them accepted cigarette advertisements, and only four had a policy of refusing cigarette advertisements. Only 31 per cent of the magazines had published an article of one page or more on smoking and health in the previous 12 months.

The tobacco industry has targeted women through campaigns that offer discounts on common household items unrelated to tobacco. Philip Morris has offered discounts on turkeys, milk, soft drinks, and laundry detergent with the purchase of tobacco products. Cigarette-branded clothing and other giveaway accessories have been used to promote cigarettes products to women and girls. Virginia Slims offered a yearly engagement calendar and the V-Wear catalogue, featuring clothing, jewellery, and accessories, coordinated the themes and colours of the print advertising with those of the product packaging. Capri Superslims used point-of-sale displays and value-added gifts featuring items such as mugs and caps bearing the Capri label in colours which coordinated with the advertisements and cigarette packaging. Misty Slims offered colour-coordinated items in multiple-pack containers. The manufacturer also offered an address book, cigarette lighter, T-shirt, and fashion booklet.

Tobacco advertising globally replicates that seen in Europe and the United States by associating smoking with success. As western-styled marketing has increased, campaigns commonly have focused on women. For example, in 1989, the brand Yves Saint Laurent introduced a new package designed to appeal to women in Malaysia and other Asian countries. National tobacco monopolies and companies, such as those in Indonesia and Japan, began to copy this promotional targeting of women.

One of the most popular media for reaching women – especially in countries where tobacco advertising is banned on TV – is women's magazines. Women's magazines are principally vehicles for promoting cosmetics, clothes and other products directed at women, including tobacco. The magazines try to lend an air of social acceptability and a stylish image to smoking. This is particularly important in countries where smoking rates are low among women and where the tobacco industry is attempting to associate smoking with Western values.

Events and activities popular among young people are often sponsored by tobacco companies. Free tickets to films and to pop and rock concerts have been given in exchange for empty cigarette packets in Hong Kong and Taiwan. Popular US female stars have allowed their names to be associated with cigarettes in other countries.

Destroying the Impact of Advertising

What can you do personally to combat the effects of tobacco advertisements? The first thing is to analyze them and see them for what they really are – a con trick designed to make a life-threatening product appear acceptable. Most advertisements are insulting and patronizing when deconstructed by careful analysis. Here is a list of some of the devices and gimmicks that historically have been directed at the unsuspecting public:

- Hide and Seek. Conceal the brand identity by using coded messages involving gold images (Benson and Hedges) or purple silk, cut by scissors or other sharp objects (Silk Cut). Children who recognize them feel that they belong to a secret society of adult consumers who are in the know about these strange and exciting hidden messages. Indirectly, these advertisements suggest to children that cigarettes are a mysterious, secretive thing, something tempting to be tried.
- Borrowed Symbols. Use a well-known image from a respectable source (for example, a puffin as used by the publisher of children's books, Puffin Books). One ad carried a picture of a puffin with its beak in the form of the corner of the gold Benson and Hedges cigarette pack. The association between smoking and the puffin symbol is strengthened by the picture of the puffin being shown as a page in a book! Another example was a construction crane decorated by Imperial Tobacco in Bristol in the UK just before Christmas

in 1991, showing Father Christmas smoking a cigar. This conveyed the vivid message that Santa thinks smoking is OK. It even implicitly suggested that children could think of giving Daddy a box of cigars for Christmas! Indirectly, this encourages young children to purchase tobacco products and to view tobacco as a happy, fun thing to buy, something that Father Christmas strongly approves of.

- Colour Associations. Here is a quick test of your recall: Which brands are associated with the following colours? (1) Gold (2) Purple (3) Black (4) Red. You probably got the first three without much difficulty. In 1991 the fourth one was still at the experimental stage. Philip Morris ran a poster campaign in Germany to promote its Marlboro brand using the slogan: 'Marlboro is Red. Red is Marlboro.' In addition to the posters, PR agents dressed in red clothing patrolled German cities during the summer and there were also red limousines, red clubs, and red buildings. Advertising is expected to be banned, and so the company presumably hopes that anything red will automatically trigger smokers to unconsciously think of Marlboro. Philip Morris clearly intended to appropriate the colour red, just as Silk Cut have already appropriated purple and Benson and Hedges the colour gold.

  Such pro-cigarette programming, in which any object of a particular colour will eventually trigger a major cigarette brand, can only be stopped by banning advertising completely. Unfortunately, before the ban is brought into force, practically every colour of the rainbow may have been given this unwanted, surplus meaning by the tobacco advertisers.

- Sexual Stereotyping. Cigarette advertising plays on the sexuality of smoking by depicting smoking as a sexy thing to do. How many movies have you seen where a couple finish making love by sharing a cigarette? How long will it be before a Hollywood director is brave enough to show a couple using a condom while making love and no cigarette afterwards?

  Films so often show the stars as people who enjoy smoking. Not only is smoking portrayed as macho, but it is projected as feminist as well. One of the most popular films of 1991 was *Thelma and Louise*, starring Susan Sarandon and Geena Davis. Following the attempted rape of one of them, Thelma and Louise hit the open road. They drank liquor out of the bottle, and constantly smoked cigarettes. *Thelma and Louise* was a box-office success. As a vivid portrayal of feminist role models, it unfortunately encouraged smoking and drinking among young women.

- Smoke and Be a Macho Marlboro Man. Like their Hollywood friends, advertisers present smoking as a tough, macho thing to do. The Marlboro cowboy is a prime example. The fact is that macho Marlboro men died of lung cancer just as quickly as anybody else. One actor who promoted Marlboro, Wayne McLaren, was a thirty-a-day smoker for 25 years before he became ill with lung cancer and died.

  Philip Morris is very possessive of its cowboy. The company sued the French health authority CFES for £1.5 million for running a TV campaign that allegedly parodied a cowboy by a campfire who stated that smoking wasn't in his nature. The court ruled in favour of the company! This provides another telling example of how a company has appropriated an image/concept that really should be nobody's to own.

- Marketing Death. 'Death' cigarettes, initially launched in California, were being sold in the UK in the 1990s. This brand was packaged in a black box with the warning: 'Cigarette smoking is addictive and debilitating. If you don't smoke, don't start. If you smoke, quit.' Each cigarette is marked with a skull and crossbones. This brand opened up new markets in record stores, which traditionally did not sell cigarettes. It is appealing to the natural risk-taking and curiosity of children and teenagers, who might be even more attracted to smoking when it is promoted as a legal but addictive drug.

- Menthol Fresh. No, not a toothpaste, but cigarettes! These long, slinky, mentholated cigarettes are all the rage in some circles. Traditionally promoted with images of mountain streams, waterfalls, and natural scenery, these tooth-staining marvels of marketing are just as harmful to health as the plain old filter brand. The con is to make the consumer think that it is possible to smoke and be healthy at the same time. This is a key strategy of the tobacco advertiser.

- Unlucky Strike. Janet Sackman, a former model for Lucky Strike and Chesterfield cigarettes in the 1940s and 1950s, was diagnosed as having cancer and became a dedicated anti-tobacco campaigner. Like Wayne McLaren, Ms Sackman unfortunately discovered the true effects of smoking the hard way. Each and every time a smoker lights a cigarette, they are one step nearer to an early death. Analyze how your ex-favourite ad tried to direct the consumer's thoughts away from the health consequences of smoking by making smoking appear attractive, sophisticated, or 'cool'.

- Cartoon Camels, Toy Money, and T-shirts. In the US, more smokers under the age of 18 smoke Camel than any other brand. In fact, there is a direct relationship between brand choice among young smokers and the amount each company spends on advertising. The company RJ Reynolds has promoted the brand using a Joe Camel cartoon character and toy money that can be cashed in for T-shirts, baseball caps, and other merchandise. Their rival company, Brown and Williamson, a subsidiary of British & American Tobacco Industries, has used a hip cartoon character called Willie, a penguin who wears sunglasses. Do you recall which ads appealed to you as a young smoker? Look at your ex-favourite ads and analyse how they were carefully designed to influence your desire to smoke.

A report published in 1991 by the Advertising Research Unit at the University of Strathclyde in Scotland proved beyond a reasonable doubt that tobacco advertising is getting through to children. Advertising encourages children who already smoke to carry on, and recruits children to smoking for the first time. Examples of children's reactions to these advertisements are best expressed in their own words, as follows:

- Hard men smoke this cigarette. . . not hard but tough, like John Wayne.
- The advertisement is telling you that if you smoke them, you're gonna be a macho he-man.
- It must be cool to smoke . . . like a cowboy . . . relaxed . . . nothing gets you going, nothing bothers you.

'Low-Tar' Cigarettes

It has been claimed by health authorities that low-tar cigarettes or 'lights' are safer and less harmful to health than higher-tar brands. Although not widely recognized, 'lights' actually contain exactly the same tobacco as ordinary high-tar brands. The only difference between high- and low-tar cigarettes is that the low-tar ones have small holes in the sides of the filters. When tar levels are measured, the concentration of tar in the smoke is lower simply because the amount of air drawn in through the filter during inhalation is higher. However, the absolute amount of tar in the smoke remains the same.

As a result of this device for producing 'lower' tar values in the official measures, there is a proportionately lower concentration of nicotine in the smoke, which provides less nicotine per puff. This entices the smoker to inhale larger puffs and/or to puff more rapidly, which in turn increases the temperature of the tobacco's combustion and produces more carbon monoxide. Carbon monoxide increases the pressure on the heart and cardiovascular system. What the smoker assumes is a safer cigarette, because of lower tar levels, is more dangerous, because the increased levels of carbon monoxide.

When smokers switch to a lower-tar brand, they experience less satisfaction, increase their consumption and inhale more deeply and/or more rapidly. In many cases new symptoms and unpleasant sensations accompany the smoker's use of the new, lower-tar brand. For example, the smoker may experience more headaches, coughs, and dryness of the throat or mouth. In some countries where low tar cigarettes have been vigorously promoted, the pack size of cigarettes was increased from 20 to 25, because manufacturers expect 20-a-day smokers to increase their consumption to 25 per day after switching to low-tar cigarettes.

Spot The Lie

What can you do to strengthen your resolve not to be taken in by cigarette marketing? One enjoyable pastime is to play 'Spot The Lie'. When you come across an ad or cigarette trigger somewhere, examine it carefully and ask what kinds of images and feelings are being linked with smoking. Of special interest is the particular brand you used to smoke.

Ads are now banned in the media in many places. But if you can find examples, from an old magazine perhaps, they could provide valuable insights into your needs and values at the time when you began to smoke cigarettes. If possible, find an old ad for the brand that you smoked. Does it suggest any of the following?

- Smoking is sexy.
- Smoking is trendy.
- Smoking is sophisticated.
- Smoking is a natural thing.
- Smokers are young and healthy.
- Smoking is associated with travel.
- Smoking is associated with excitement.
- Smoking is associated with images of success.
- Smoking is associated with images of luxury.
- Smoking is associated with images of wealth (for example, silver and gold).

Analyse the content of some advertisements for your former favourite brand. Remember that each advertisement is the end product of millions of pounds of investment. Destroy it mentally by analysing it.

Tobacco Sponsorship

Sponsorship of sport and the arts is linked with the tobacco advertisers' images of health, taking a safe risk, and excitement. More upscale, trendy sports – such as motor racing, tennis, or golf – are favoured by the tobacco sponsors, but, pool, and darts have also been sponsored. Arts and music events, such as jazz festivals, art exhibitions and competitions, also accept sponsorship from tobacco companies.

Sponsorship of sporting and arts events is carefully planned to have the maximum possible impact on new smokers. The appeal to young people, particularly through motor racing, is very strong. In the US, tobacco advertising has been banned from radio and television since 1971, but the TV presence of tobacco products remains highly significant in spite of the ban. In a single 94-minute car race (the Marlboro Grand Prix), Marlboro was seen or mentioned 5,993 times, for a total of 46 minutes. This is equivalent to $1 million of free airtime!

The tobacco industry claims that banning their sponsorship would lead to the collapse of many key sports and cultural events but there is no reason why this needs to happen. However, sports bodies are confident that they could find new sponsors for their major events to cover the 10% of income currently drawn from the tobacco industry. When sponsorship was banned in Australia in 1996, sponsorship of sport actually *increased* following a tobacco ban. The association of cigarette advertising with prestigious cultural and sporting events lends credibility and respectability to the industry and to cigarette smoking. This is another reason why all forms of tobacco sponsorship must be completely banned as soon as possible.

Tobacco's sponsorship of world sport extends across every continent, from kart racing in Columbia to Uganda's 'Sportsman of the Year' award, sponsored by British American Tobacco's Sportsman brand.

Diversification

Tobacco companies are seeking to advertise cigarettes indirectly. They have started trading in luxury goods to promote their brands by selling expensive, high-quality clothing, accessories, cigarette lighters, and other items. This marketing strategy will enable the companies to establish themselves in other markets and retain their visibility on the main shopping streets.

All kinds of businesses are likely to start popping up as fronts for the tobacco companies. One example was a 'travel company' advertising under a well known cigarette brand name in Malaysia. When holiday seekers tried to book their holidays, they were told that there were none available or they were referred to the main office in another country. As and when a full advertising ban becomes law, all kinds of 'diversification' will occur where the familiar tobacco names will appear on new kinds of products which can be lawfully advertised. A truly effective advertising ban would have to include indirect advertising, but that seems unlikely to happen on technical grounds.

Litigation

Tobacco litigation punishes the tobacco industry for its misconduct and deceit – whether on health damage or smuggling. Litigation has forced the disclosure of 35 million pages of secret documents revealing the industry's strategic approach to hiding the truth about tobacco. On 24 June 1992, the American Supreme Court ruled that health warnings on cigarette packets do not protect manufacturers from being sued by people suffering from smoking-related diseases. This resulted in a series of lawsuits against cigarette companies who have denied that smoking causes disease and death. For decades, tobacco companies have deceived the public about the dangers of smoking by hiding their research findings showing how harmful tobacco can be.

The Supreme Court decision opened the door to people with

smoking-related diseases to claim that they had not been sufficiently warned about the specific dangers and risk levels associated with smoking. This historic decision forced the tobacco companies either to publicly admit that smoking causes disease and death, or to defend themselves in court against plaintiffs who allege that the companies have sent out confusing messages about the hazards of smoking.

Litigation in the USA has been on an enormous scale. The major tobacco companies are having to defend hundreds of cases. As of 31 December 2001, the British firm British American Tobacco had 4,419 product liability cases pending against it.

The first class action on behalf of smokers to go to trial was in Florida, the so-called 'Engle Case', named after a paediatrician who contracted emphysema. Howard Engle claimed damages on behalf of 40,000 to 50,000 Florida residents made ill through smoking. In July 1999, the jury found tobacco manufacturers guilty of making an addictive and defective product, and for conspiring to hide the dangers of smoking. The industry was also found potentially liable for punitive damages.

On 3 September 1999, a Florida appeals court ruled that any damages claims in the class action would have to be assessed one smoker at a time. This was considered a victory for the tobacco firms, because it removed the possibility that they would be hit by a massive punitive damage award, which could have ranged from £200 to £500 billion. The jury awarded $6.9 million in compensatory damages to lung cancer victim Mary Farnan and to a widower whose wife had died of lung cancer in the summer of 1999, aged 53. Huge damages could bankrupt the industry. The Florida legislature passed a bill limiting the amount of any bond to $100 million or 10 per cent of the tobacco companies' net worth, whichever is the lower.

Another massive case has been brought by the US Federal Government. On 22 September 1999, the United States Justice Department filed a multi-billion-dollar lawsuit to recoup money spent by the government on health care for smoking-related illnesses. The lawsuit was intended to force the industry to finance smoking education and cessation programmes. The federal government spends approximately $20 billion a year treating smoking-related diseases, and statutes of limitations permit the government to go back three years to recover costs under the Medical Care Recovery Act and six years under the Medicare law governing health payments for the elderly. The former US Attorney General, Janet Reno, said: 'For more than 45 years, the cigarette companies conducted their business without regard to the truth, the law, or the health of the American people.'

In 1999 the first group action in the UK was concluded. Fifty-two people with lung cancer sued two British tobacco companies, Gallaher and Imperial Tobacco, but the case was overturned on legal technicalities. The judge had ruled that 36 of the lung cancer sufferers could not continue their case against the companies because they had been diagnosed with the disease more than three years before suing. Lord Justice Wright ruled that the majority of the plaintiffs were time-barred, and so the plaintiffs' lawyers decided that the risks of pursuing the case with so few remaining plaintiffs were too great.

A London croupier, Micky Dunn, is suing his employers after suffering attacks of asthma which Dunn claims were caused by the casino's smoky atmosphere. A mother who claimed that passive smoking affected her unborn child's health has won a battle for compensation. Colette Comstive's son, Matthew, suffered from asthma and recurring chest infections after she was forced to work in a smoky office during her pregnancy. After a four-year battle, the boy was awarded £5,000 and £5,800 costs.

Fifty bar workers in Ireland are suing their employers and the tobacco industry, having suffered illnesses including emphysema and lung cancer, claiming that they were harmed directly as a result of smoking and indirectly by their working environment.

In Italy, two bank managers based in Milan have been found guilty of manslaughter, following the death of an employee who was exposed to tobacco smoke. A 35-year old woman with severe asthma was forced to work in a smoky environment, despite frequent written requests to move to a cleaner environment. She collapsed and died of an acute asthma attack, after months of working in a small, windowless office with habitual smokers.

In the Netherlands, a court ruled that employers must guarantee that non-smoking staff will have a working environment completely free from tobacco smoke. The Breda district court upheld a postal worker's complaint that exposure to tobacco smoke at the city's sorting office infringed on her right to work in a smoke-free environment.

In the US, a class-action lawsuit by a group of casino workers was settled in June 2002. About 1,000 current and former employees of a New Orleans riverboat casino will receive $2.6 million in compensation for ailments caused by passive smoking. The suit claimed that employees suffered respiratory illnesses ranging from occupational asthma to sinusitis, bronchitis and other infections and ailments, some of which were severe enough to require hospitalization.

A new development has been the filing of lawsuits against tobacco companies for misleading consumers about the health impact of 'light' or low-tar cigarettes. As pointed out above, any supposed benefits of smoking a low-tar cigarette are cancelled out by the smoker's deeper and harder inhalations. During the last couple of years, tobacco companies have begun putting information about this compensation phenomenon on their Websites. A few companies also print a small disclaimer in their ads, noting that tar and nicotine intake vary with the way people smoke. However, industry documents have revealed that the companies were aware of the phenomenon more than thirty years ago.

In March 2002, a jury in Portland, Oregon ordered Philip Morris to pay $168,000 in damages and $150 million in punitive damages to the estate of a woman who smoked the company's low-tar Merit brand. Michelle Schwartz died from lung cancer at the age of 53. The jury found that Philip Morris had made false claims to the effect that light cigarettes were less harmful than regular brands. The jury also found that the company's Merit cigarettes were 'defective and unreasonably dangerous'. Similar cases are pending in a dozen states and are expected to be filed in others.

Summary

- Think about your reactions to cigarette marketing. Analyse how you were deceived by ads when you were a smoker.
- Decide how you will respond to cigarette marketing in the future.
- Think about your general attitude towards the commercial and political aspects of the tobacco industry. What can you do to activate public opinion against cigarette advertising?
- Write to organizations receiving sponsorship from the tobacco industry encouraging them to look for alternative sponsors.
- Make sure that anybody you know who is still a smoker is fully informed about the true facts about 'lights'/low-tar cigarettes.
- In light of what you know about the marketing of cigarettes, harden your resolve never to smoke cigarettes again.

In November 2004 the UK Government announced that it is considering a ban on smoking in public places in England. It could follow in the footsteps of Norway and Ireland and introduce a nationwide smoking ban or it could just give more powers to councils allowing them to introduce local bans. Also Scotland voted to introduce a smoking ban in enclosed public places. The ban will come into force from Spring 2006.

12

Life Skills for the Ex-smoker – Finally Quitting for Life

This final chapter focuses on the psychological aspects of becoming a successful non-smoker. You have the awareness and skills necessary for coping with the traps and pitfalls that may be set by others. However, anybody who tries to break your resolve by tempting you with cigarettes, or giving you a hard time, is really on the defensive. You need to be in charge and make your own choices, rather than have them imposed on you by other people and events.

It is important at this stage to develop your strategies for minimizing the risk of relapse. Some of the more significant, longer-term factors in changing your lifestyle have been covered in the preceding chapters. You also need to be on your guard against momentary slips or lapses that could take you unawares, and push you back into your earlier groove of smoking. To help you avoid this, here is a list of the key danger points.

Preventing Relapse

The biggest task for the ex-smoker is preventing lapses or slips. A considerable amount of research in recent years has been directed towards the identification of situations where slips are most likely to occur. This is because any single slip can potentially lead to a full-blown relapse and it is therefore necessary to be on the alert for high-risk situations. The major danger-points are:

- Negative emotional states and mood swings: frustration, anxiety, depression, boredom, or loneliness. Ways of coping with these moods swings and feelings without smoking, eating, or drinking are described in some detail in Chapter nine.
- Positive emotional states: success, joy, happiness, and good company. Fortunately, you're less likely to lapse when you're in a positive mood than when you're in a negative mood, but lapses can still happen. All that can really be said here is: don't spoil it by smoking.
- Social pressure: this can be direct, for example when somebody offers you a cigarette; or indirect, for example when you're in the company of smokers at a party, and you end up asking somebody for a cigarette. This is discussed in more detail on page 190 below.
- Conflict/stress: this can occur almost anywhere but the key situations are at work and at home. Forty to fifty per cent of all relapses are attributed to stress of various kinds, so you must learn to deal with stressful situations without relying on a cigarette. Suggestions about how to do this are provided in Chapter eight. It will also help you if you remember and understand some of the basic characteristics of smokers.

Understanding Smokers

You can easily understand smokers because only recently you were one! You could even admit that you still are a potential smoker. Smokers are one of the biggest external influences on your success or failure, but only if you let them be. Some smokers may even attempt to sabotage your best efforts to remain a non-smoker, and you need to be prepared to deal with them. You have successfully completed the first stage of becoming a non-smoker and it is vital that you remain a non-smoker for the rest of your life. You can achieve this in spite of Pro-Cigarette Programs (PCPs) or smokers trying to backslide you out of your non-smoking groove into your old groove as a smoker. The power of your very much weakened PCPs, which could still be lying dormant somewhere inside your biocomputer, needs to be continually monitored, as does the potential influence of smokers you run into in everyday life. The way you deal with them could make all the difference to your long-term success.

For many, smoking is a key part of their life, a tool for changing bad moods into good, for relaxing or activating, and for a hundred other momentary purposes. Smoking accompanies practically everything that the smoker does from the first to the last waking moment each day, and permeates everything the smoker comes into contact with, thinks about or has a feeling about. Stopping and starting things, having a conversation, eating, drinking, thinking, or simply doing nothing in particular, are all associated with smoking. In some cases, smokers will go to incredible lengths to keep cigarette smoke in their lungs.

The city where I once lived in New Zealand, Dunedin, is situated at the end of a beautiful harbour. For several miles, the road runs right beside the sea, only a few feet below. One summer, three different smokers drove into the harbour as a result of dropping lit cigarettes between their legs onto the driver's seat!

I once met a lung surgeon who had spent 30 years removing lungs and tumours from patients suffering from one of the worst and most painful conditions caused by smoking, lung cancer. I could hardly believe it when the surgeon took out a packet of cigarettes, offered me one, and admitted that he was a 25-a-day smoker!

Many smokers are almost totally dominated by the quest for nicotine, and the majority like to smoke in company whenever possible. Doing something in a crowd makes it feel more acceptable. You need to be constantly on guard because the smoker may strike when you least expect it. Watch out for the 'feel good' factor, when you feel as if you can cope with anything. Smoking and drinking tend to go together and so you will be most at risk in situations where alcohol flows.

Something like 50 to 60 per cent of all lapses occur as a result of obtaining a cigarette from another smoker. In many cases the lapse occurs while alcohol, food, tea or coffee are being consumed, and smokers just fall back into their old ways. As an ex-smoker, you may not behave or think rationally, as far as your smoking is concerned, for several months or years following quitting. Once a smoker you are always a smoker, potentially. Your smoking friends may therefore unwittingly put you at risk simply by smoking in your company. One key to successful relapse prevention is to learn to manage social situations where eating and drinking occurs in the company of smokers.

Assertiveness

So how should you handle smokers if they try to reconvert you to their cause? You need to listen carefully to what they say but, if necessary, treat it with a pinch of salt. Assert your right to not smoke. Smokers need to accept and respect your views too.

The key concept to remember is that you and you alone are in charge of your mind and body. Assert this right whenever there is any doubt about the matter. Assert your right not to smoke and not to inhale passively the smoke of others.

One of the most important, and yet complex, issues to deal with is smoking at your place of work. If your workplace is not already smoke-free, you should raise the issue with your manager and ask for a smoke-free policy. This will require a survey of staff opinion throughout the organization, in order to establish new rules about smoking in the workplace. Smokers will need to be given a smoking zone, isolated from smoke-free areas, where smoking will be permitted during agreed times, such as coffee breaks and lunch breaks. Open-plan offices will need to be made completely smokeless, as will cafeterias and all other communal spaces. Eventually smoking within the office environment will be phased out completely, so your company or organization will be smoke-free.

Managing Time

For many people, life seems to be speeding up, so there is little time to plan or think or 'chill out'. Everybody these days is talking about stress – the stress of working, the stress of commuting, stress from the family, or simply the stress of living – but it is an abused and misapplied term which is rarely ever properly defined. Everybody thinks that they automatically know what stress is. However, it is a term that even so-called 'experts' often do not define in any clear or meaningful way.

Most uses of the term 'stress' would be better served by the term 'strain', following the original concepts in engineering. Strain is what occurs in an object when stresses are placed upon it. Thus the stress of a hurricane may cause too great a strain on a busy suspension bridge and lead to its collapse. 'Stress' is a property of the hurricane (the surrounding environment) and 'strain' a property of the bridge (the human being).

Recent theories have looked at the relationship between the resources of a person and the demands placed on those resources in the course of everyday living. When a person's resources are insufficient to meet the demands placed upon them, strain is the inevitable result. A person's resources consist of everything they have for the process of living, whether material, in the form of money and tangible assets; or psychological, in the form of knowledge, abilities and skills; or social, in the form of support from family, friends, and colleagues at work. All three factors contribute to making as big a change as quitting smoking for life.

One of the most important resources is time. Like any other, it is finite and the way it is used can prevent, or provoke, strain. By carefully planning how you use your time, you will have more control over your wellbeing. One of the greatest stressors is having too little time to finish the things that you believe that you need to get done. Managing time is therefore closely linked with your ability to say no. When excessive demands are placed upon you, whether at work or at home, you need to be clear about what you can and cannot manage in the time available. This requires sitting down and planning carefully how long each task is going to take and how many other things you need to do within a particular timescale. The thing to remember is that we practically always underestimate how long things really do take. A good rule of thumb is to add 50 per cent to the time you allow to do things, just to be on the safe side of the stress-strain equation.

One of the most effective ways of reducing strain is to take on only those things that you know you can complete within the time available. Timetables are therefore essential. If you don't have one already, buy a diary which has enough space to plan your days by the hour. Sit down with your diary and plan when and where you are going and what you are going to do. Leave days free for essential things you know you normally have a problem fitting in. Cancel or postpone activities that are of low priority and things that you know you cannot fit in. Always allow enough time for any necessary preparation and for any follow-up activities that may be required afterwards (e.g. reports, letters, emails, telephone calls, or for just letting everything 'gel').

Time management has a lot to do with privacy, and not being available at certain times so that you can attend to your own needs for relaxation and care, both mental and physical. Routines are very helpful, so that others can learn when you will be available for certain activities and when you will be unavailable. Accessibility is a key factor. If you have never thought about these issues before, now would be an excellent time to take stock of what your duties, responsibilities, and needs really are. When you have considered them carefully, you will want to negotiate with others who might be affected by what the new 'accessibility' rules are going to be. Others among family, friends and colleagues will need to adjust their expectations and timetables accordingly.

Your preferences may sometimes conflict with those of others, so you will need to negotiate a way of dealing with the problem. Aim at a compromise which leaves everybody feeling happy about what is planned for your future time together. Give yourself the best chance of minimizing avoidable strains resulting from poor time management.

Relaxation

One of your best long-term strategies as a confirmed non-smoker will be to ensure you have plenty of relaxation. Make relaxation a central part of your daily, weekly, and monthly routines. As a non-smoker you will have more money, more time, and more energy. Why not develop a new interest or pastime to enhance your enjoyment of life and promote relaxation?

As we saw in Chapter nine, physical leisure activities can provide an important source of relaxation as the mind is given the chance to take itself away from everyday worries and concerns. It doesn't really matter which form of relaxation you choose but, if you can combine mental relaxation with physical activity, it will be even more beneficial.

Controlling Stress and Strain

Stress, strain, and how to control them has become almost a new religion. For many people the Sunday paper, magazines and TV have replaced the Sunday sermon as a source of advice on how to live; psychologists, counsellors, and doctors are replacing the local priest as exorcists of this late twentieth-century obsession. However, you have the greatest power to reduce the strain in your life.

As a non-smoker, you have taken control of your body from the automatic programming which kept you smoking. This major change symbolizes a whole new approach to your ways of dealing and coping with stress and strain. It gives you a completely new self-image in which you make the decisions about your life. Smoking had become a source of great stress to you, but that is now in your past. This programme has provided you with a powerful set of methods which you can use to eliminate many of the other stresses that you will encounter in your everyday life.

Although people who lapse into smoking give many different reasons for restarting the habit, 'stress' is by far the most common. This can take the form of unexpected or tragic life events, such as accidents, deaths, or family illnesses; or it may consist of arguments, separations, divorces, redundancies, or other events which pose a major threat to personal security. These events are often unpredicted, unplanned, and unrehearsed. You therefore need to build up your personal reserves so that you are better equipped to deal with any potential threat. You can build up your reserves using all of the methods suggested in Part Two of this book. Greater physical fitness toughens you both physically and mentally. If you are worried about your weight, learning to control your eating habits and taking more exercise will help you to correct the problem. Relaxation, better time management, and being better able to assert your rights and preferences are three other key strategies for protecting yourself from avoidable strain. The methods described in this book provide you with health protective behaviours for the future enhancement of your wellbeing.

One of the greatest factors is the power of your thinking to influence the way you see things in the first place. This is really the old division between pessimists and optimists. 'For there is nothing either good or bad but thinking makes it so.' Today, psychologists are investigating how the explanations people give for the events in their lives reflect optimistic or pessimistic thinking styles. While optimists treat stress as a challenge and live to fight another day, pessimists see almost everything as a problem and find everything simply too much to cope with.

Stress and strain can never be eliminated altogether. In fact, a life without challenges would be very dull indeed. What we can all learn to do better is not to allow unavoidable events to immobilize us, blocking the creative processes of growth, development, and recovery. The next chapter in life's unfolding story is always there waiting to begin. The success that you achieve in quitting smoking for life hopefully will make a positive contribution to your physical wellbeing and to your self-belief. Psychologists refer to this as 'self-efficacy'. Using the tools provided by this programme, you can successfully change your behaviour. The various methods that have been described are easy to apply and quite general in their application. If you have applied them systematically to your smoking behaviour, and continue to do so, you can give yourself an excellent chance of successfully quitting for life. You should also be able to adapt the methods to achieve other objectives in your life. In this way, you can make further improvements in your physical, psychological, and social wellbeing. The mind is the most powerful instrument we have. If this programme has helped you to use your mind to improve your physical health, it will have succeeded.

Summary

- Be on your guard against high-risk situations.
- Assert your right not to smoke and not to breathe other people's smoke.
- Learn to manage your time as efficiently as possible so that you are less pressured by other people and events.
- Set aside time on a regular basis purely for your own relaxation.
- Develop a new interest or hobby to add to the quality of your life.
- Manage stress by preventing it to begin with.
- Remain as positive as possible: 'for there is nothing either good or bad but thinking makes it so'.
- Live and enjoy your new life to the full!

Abbreviations

ACPs – Anti-Cigarette Programs
CBT – cognitive behavior therapy
CHD – coronary heart disease
COPD – chronic obstructive pulmonary disease
ETS – environmental tobacco smoke
MAO – monoamineoxidase
MDS – mesolimbic dopamine system
NO – Nitrous oxide
NRT – Nicotine replacement therapy
PCPs – Pro-Cigarette Programs
PPCAs – Phoney Pro-Cigarette Arguments
QFL – Quit for Life
SCOTH – the Scientific Committee on Smoking and Health
SIDS – Sudden Infant Death Syndrome
WHO – World Health Organization
WOT – withdrawal-oriented therapy

Useful References

Government Reports on Smoking

Report of the Scientific Committee on Tobacco and Health, Department of Health. London: The Stationery Office, 1998. See also: http://www.archive.official-documents.co.uk/document/doh/tobacco/report.htm

US Department of Health & Human Services, *Clinical practice guideline 18: Smoking cessation.* Washington DC: US Government Printing Office,(Agency for health care policy and reseach; publication no 96-0692), 1996. See also: http://www.guideline.gov/summary/summary.aspx?ss=15&doc_id=2360&string=

Surgeon General, *The Health Consequences of Smoking: A Report of the Surgeon General,* Washington, USA: Office of the Surgeon General, 2004. See also: http://www.surgeon general.gov/library/smokingconsequences/

References on the CBT Approach to Quitting

Gordon Marlatt and Judith Gordon (Eds), *Relapse Prevention: Maintenance Strategies in the Treatment of Addictive Behavior,* New York: Guilford Press, 1985.

David F. Marks, Smoking cessation as a test-bed for psychological theory: a group cognitive therapy programme with high long-term abstinence rates. *Journal of Smoking-Related Disorders,* 1992, 3, 69–78.

David F. Marks, Addiction, smoking and health: Developing policy-based interventions, *Psychology, Health & Medicine*, 1998, 3, 97–111.

Catherine M Sykes and David F. Marks, Effectiveness of a cognitive behaviour therapy self-help programme for smokers in London, UK. *Health Promotion International*, 2001, 16, 255–260.

David F. Marks and Catherine M. Sykes, A randomized controlled trial of cognitive behaviour therapy for smokers living in a deprived part of London, *Psychology, Health & Medicine*, 2002, 7, 17–24.

David F. Marks & Catherine M. Sykes, Cognitive behaviour therapy for smokers. Chapter 4 in *A Clinician's Guide to Behavioural Medicine: A Case Formulation Approach*, Edited by Andrzej R. Kuczmierczyk & Ana V. Nikcevik. Brunner-Routledge, 2004.

References on the NRT Approach to Quitting

Silagy C., Lancaster T., Stead L., Mant D., Fowler G., Nicotine replacement therapy for smoking cessation (Cochrane Review). In: *The Cochrane Library*, Issue 2. Chichester, UK: John Wiley & Sons, Ltd., 2004. See also: http://www.cochrane.org/resources/brochure.htm

National Institute for Clinical Excellence, Guidance on the use of nicotine replacement therapy (NRT) and bupropion for smoking cessation, Technology Appraisal Guidance No. 39, March 2002. See also: http://www.nice.org.uk/page.aspx?o=30631

Other Self-Help Books Supporting Quitting

Lowell Kleinman and Deborah Messina-Kleinman, *Complete Idiot's Guide to Quitting Smoking*, Alpha Books, 2000.

David Brizer, *Quitting Smoking For Dummies*, For Dummies, 2003.

Edwin B. Fisher, *American Lung Association 7-Steps To A Smoke-Free Life*, Wiley, 1998.

Richard Craze, *The Voice of Tobacco: A Dedicated Smoker's Diary of Not Smoking*, White Ladder Press, 2003.

Other Useful Self-Help Books Tackling Issues Relevant to Quitting Smoking

Wayne W. Dyer, *Your Erroneous Zones*, HarperTorch, Reissue edition 1997.

Wayne W. Dyer, *Pulling Your Own Strings*, HarperTorch, Reprint edition, 1994.

Ian Robertson and Nick Heather, *Let's Drink To Your Health! A Self-Help Guide To Sensible Drinking*. Leicester: BPS Books, 1986.

Melanie Fennell, *Overcoming Low Self-Esteem*, Constable, 1999.

Jan Scott, *Overcoming Mood Swings*, Constable, 2001.

Helen Kennerley, *Overcoming Anxiety*, Constable, 1997.

Appendix A
Progress Chart (Smoking)

Use this Chart to monitor your progress until you reach your D-Day. Your consumption should be added to the Progress Chart at the end of each 24-hour period.

Appendix A

PROGRESS CHART (SMOKING)

Use this Chart to monitor your progress until you reach your D-Day. It shows the reduction in consumption which has been obtained using this Programme. Your consumption should be added to the Progress Chart at the end of each 24-hour period. Note that the scale is measured in percentages of your original consumption level.

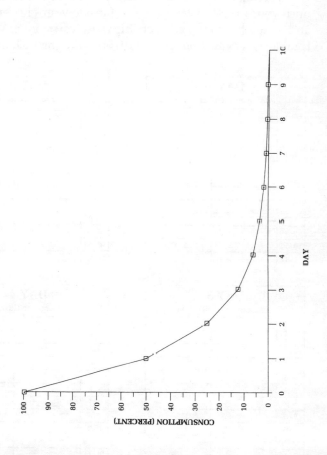

Appendix B
Daily Reduction 'Cards'

Use the 'cards' printed on this page and the next page to record every cigarette, or part of a cigarette, you smoke during the Programme. It is recommended that you photocopy the page and cut out the cards with a pair of scissors. Please use a new card each day to cover a 24-hour period. The 9 cards will last until your D-Day. Keep each card inside your cigarette packet and remember to record every cigarette you smoke. Write your total for every 24-hour period on your Progress Chart.

DAY 1	a.m. NURD p.m.	
12–1		
1–2		
2–3		
3–4		
4–5		
5–6		
6–7		
7–8		
8–9		
9–10		
10–11		
11–12		

DAY 2	a.m. NURD p.m.	
12–1		
1–2		
2–3		
3–4		
4–5		
5–6		
6–7		
7–8		
8–9		
9–10		
10–11		
11–12		

DAY 3	a.m. NURD p.m.	
12–1		
1–2		
2–3		
3–4		
4–5		
5–6		
6–7		
7–8		
8–9		
9–10		
10–11		
11–12		

DAY 4	a.m. NURD p.m.	
12–1		
1–2		
2–3		
3–4		
4–5		
5–6		
6–7		
7–8		
8–9		
9–10		
10–11		
11–12		

DAY 5 a.m. NURD p.m.		
12–1		
1–2		
2–3		
3–4		
4–5		
5–6		
6–7		
7–8		
8–9		
9–10		
10–11		
11–12		

DAY 6 a.m. NURD p.m.		
12–1		
1–2		
2–3		
3–4		
4–5		
5–6		
6–7		
7–8		
8–9		
9–10		
10–11		
11–12		

DAY 7 a.m. NURD p.m.		
12–1		
1–2		
2–3		
3–4		
4–5		
5–6		
6–7		
7–8		
8–9		
9–10		
10–11		
11–12		

DAY 8 a.m. NURD p.m.		
12–1		
1–2		
2–3		
3–4		
4–5		
5–6		
6–7		
7–8		
8–9		
9–10		
10 11		
11–12		

DAY 9 a.m. NURD p.m.		
12–1		
1–2		
2–3		
3–4		
4–5		
5–6		
6–7		
7–8		
8–9		
9–10		
10–11		
11–12		

Appendix C
Progress Chart (Eating)

Use this Progress Chart to monitor your success in keeping to your Personal Eating Rules. Write the three techniques you decided to use in the space provided below and at the end of every 24–hour period give yourself a rating from 1 to 5 for how well you applied each of the techniques.

5 = Very Well, 4 = Well, 3 = Average, 2 = Poorly, 1 = Very Poorly.

(1) _____

(2) _____

(3) _____

Day	1st Technique	2nd Technique	3rd Technique
1	[ ]	[ ]	[ ]
2	[ ]	[ ]	[ ]
3	[ ]	[ ]	[ ]
4	[ ]	[ ]	[ ]
5	[ ]	[ ]	[ ]
6	[ ]	[ ]	[ ]
7	[ ]	[ ]	[ ]
8	[ ]	[ ]	[ ]
9	[ ]	[ ]	[ ]
10	[ ]	[ ]	[ ]
11	[ ]	[ ]	[ ]
12	[ ]	[ ]	[ ]
13	[ ]	[ ]	[ ]
14	[ ]	[ ]	[ ]

15	[ ]	[ ]	[ ]
16	[ ]	[ ]	[ ]
17	[ ]	[ ]	[ ]
18	[ ]	[ ]	[ ]
19	[ ]	[ ]	[ ]
20	[ ]	[ ]	[ ]
21	[ ]	[ ]	[ ]
22	[ ]	[ ]	[ ]
23	[ ]	[ ]	[ ]
24	[ ]	[ ]	[ ]
25	[ ]	[ ]	[ ]
26	[ ]	[ ]	[ ]
27	[ ]	[ ]	[ ]
28	[ ]	[ ]	[ ]

RULES FOR SNACKING

Write your personal Rules for Snacking in the spaces below

WHERE:

WHEN:

WHAT:

Give yourself a rating from 1 to 5 at the end of every 24-hour period, for how well you applied your Rules for Snacking:
5 = Very Well, 4 = Well, 3 = Average, 2 = Poorly, 1 = Very Poorly.

DAYS

1   2   3   4   5   6   7   8   9   10   11   12   13   14

DAYS

15   16   17   18   19   20   21   22   23   24   25   26   27   28

EATING TRIGGERS

1   _____

2   _____

3   _____

4   _____

5   _____

6   _____

7   _____

8   _____

9   _____

10 _____

Appendix D
Useful Websites

These Websites are all concerned with smoking, tobacco control and quitting.

They may be helpful if you require particular kinds of information.

Action on Smoking and Health (ASH)

ASH is a charity set up in 1971 by the Royal College of Physicians in London to alert the public to the dangers of smoking and so prevent the disease, disability and death it causes.
http://www.ash.org.uk/

Centers for Disease Control and Prevention

The Centers for Disease Control and Prevention (CDC) is the lead federal agency for protecting health and safety and is the national centre for developing and applying disease prevention and control, environmental health, and health promotion and education activities designed to improve the health of the people in the United States.
http://www.cdc.gov/

National Institute on Drug Abuse

The National Institute on Drug Abuse (NIDA) in the US supports over 85 per cent of the world's research on the health aspects of drug abuse and addiction. NIDA supported science addresses fundamental questions about drug abuse, including smoking.
http://www.nida.nih.gov/

Surgeon General

The US Surgeon General reports to the Assistant Secretary for Health, who is the principal advisor to the Secretary on public health and scientific issues. The Surgeon General has provided many comprehensive and evidence-based reports on smoking and health.

http://www.surgeongeneral.gov/library/smokingconsequences/

Index

Index

Index

Index

Index